INTERMITTENT FASTING

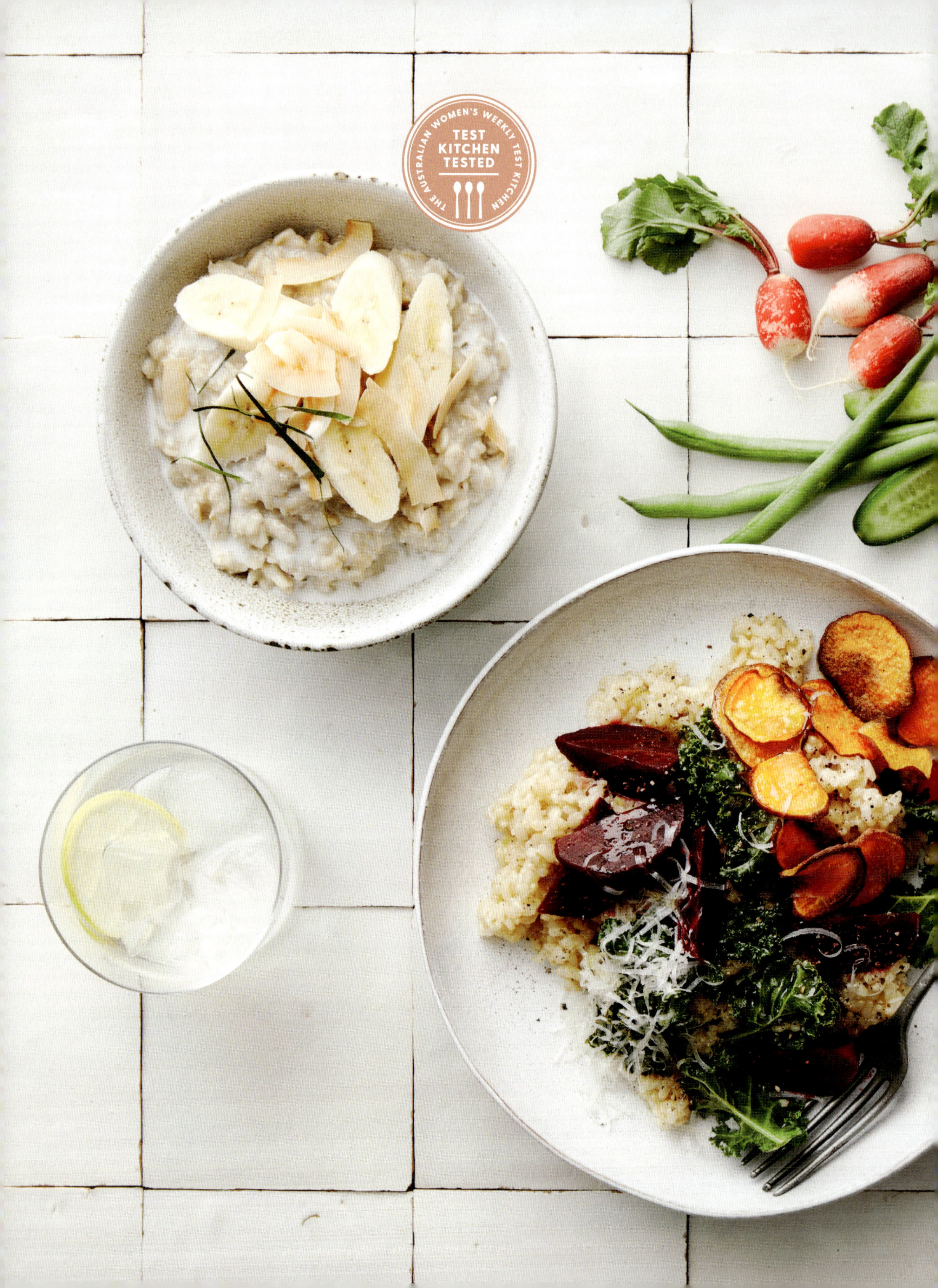
THE AUSTRALIAN WOMEN'S WEEKLY TEST KITCHEN
TEST
KITCHEN
TESTED

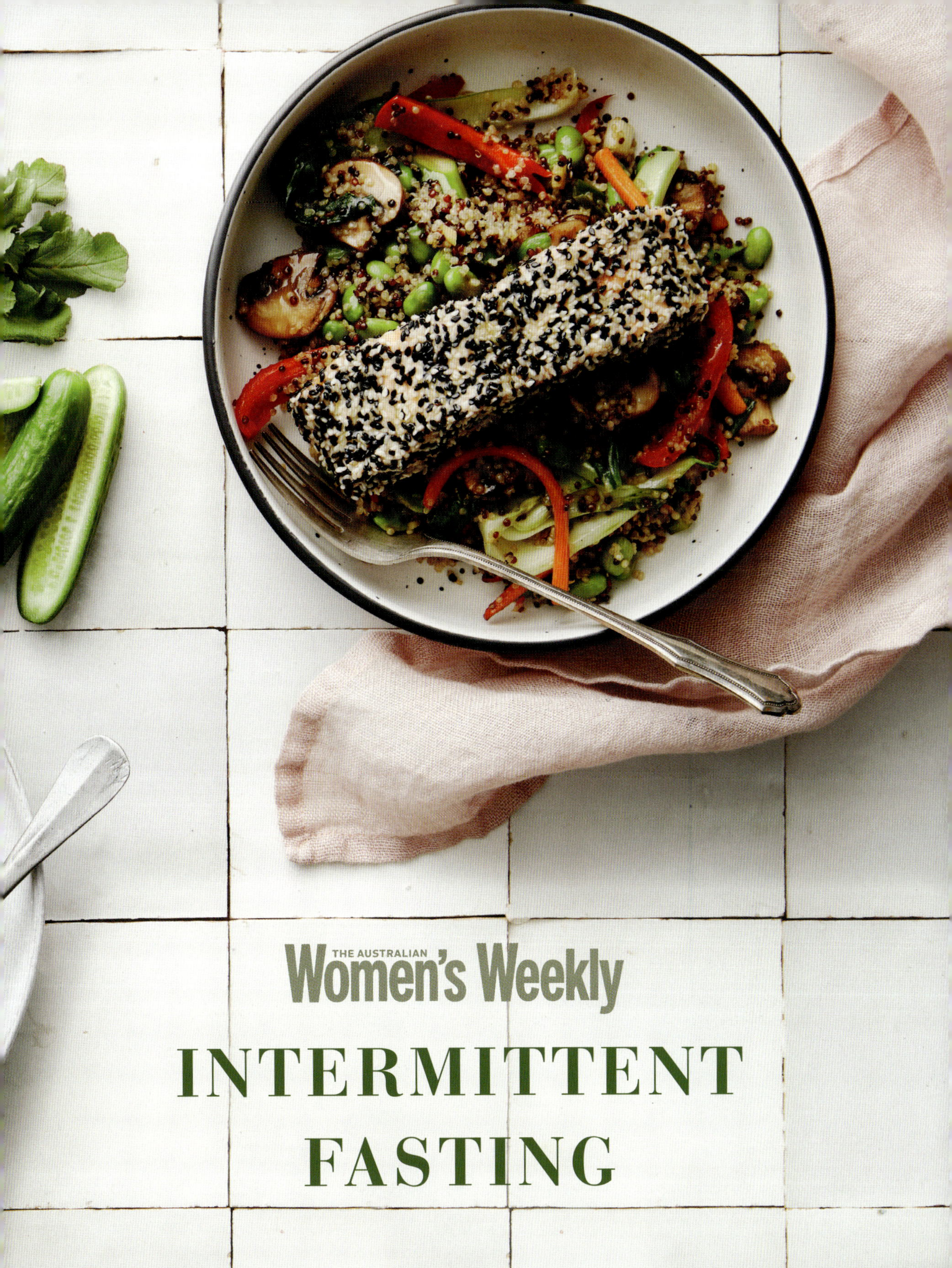

THE AUSTRALIAN
Women's Weekly

INTERMITTENT FASTING

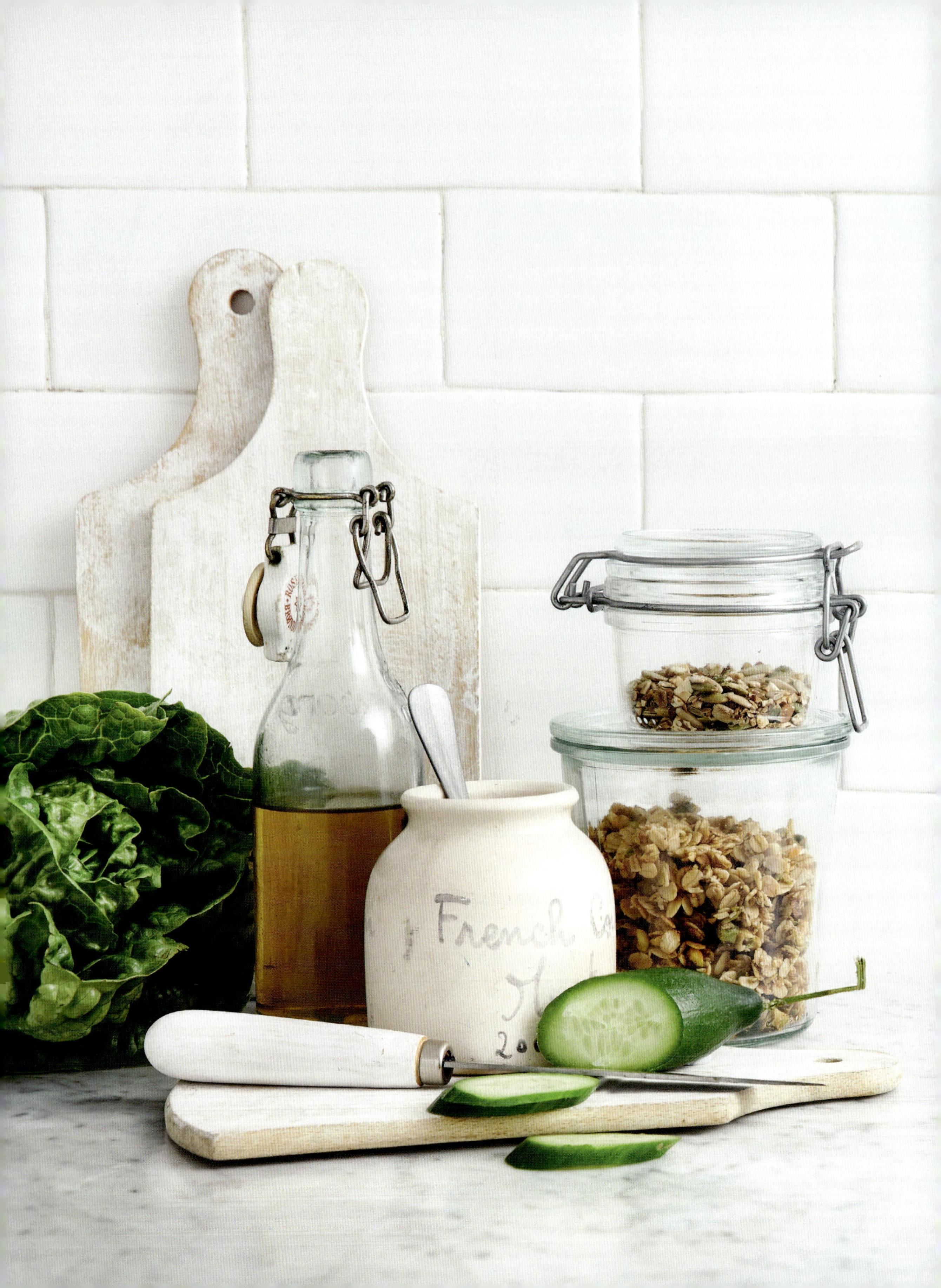
French

CONTENTS

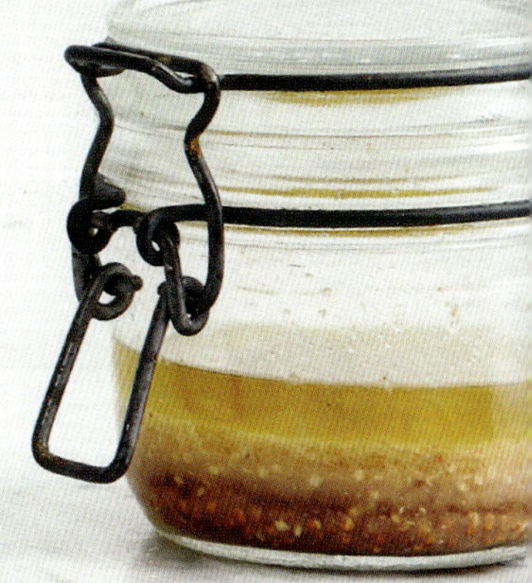

HOW TO FAST

What if we told you, you could lose weight and maintain a healthy social life without cutting out on all the foods you love? Well, you can! Intermittent fasting might sound like a miracle, but here's how it really works...

WHAT IS INTERMITTENT FASTING?

Intermittent fasting is restricting your energy intake to certain periods of the day or prolonging fasting intervals between meals, in order to extend the amount of time where our bodies are in the important rest and repair mode.

For most of us, intermittent fasting is known purely as a way to achieve our weight loss goals. While this is true, there are many other benefits as well. Recent studies show it can provide anti-inflammatory effects, improve cell health, decrease blood pressure, and even support brain and gut health.

Intermittent fasting also offers major benefits for insulin resistance and can lead to an impressive reduction in blood sugar levels, especially for men. Some studies have shown a reduction in blood sugar levels by a massive 20-31% and a reduction in fasting blood sugar by 3-6%!

Intermittent fasting also offers major benefits for insulin resistance and can lead to an impressive reduction in blood sugar levels.

HOW DOES IT WORK?

Generally speaking, when attempting to use intermittent fasting to lose weight, you naturally tend to create an energy deficit simply because you've shortened the time when you're allowed to eat.

Additionally, the activation of our body's rest and repair mode allows our body to focus on using more of our stored energy supplies so that we burn off fat and lose weight.

It causes a change in hormone levels which make stored body fat more accessible to us. This is where the magic of intermittent fasting takes place!

Thanks to the effects of intermittent fasting on your hormones, this way of eating actually increases your metabolic rate by 3.6-14%, helping you burn even more energy.

When we allow adequate time for our body to rest between meals, our bodies begin ***important cellular repair processes*** *that kickstart other health benefits too.*

HOW DO I DO IT?

There are a variety of ways you can practise intermittent fasting. Some people choose a 24-hour fast on alternate days, or a fast two days per week on non-consecutive days.

However, one of the most common ways follows a 16:8 principle, where you give yourself a daily window of 8 hours to consume your meals.

This style of intermittent fasting works because you can choose when to have your 8-hour window according to the time that best suits your schedule. For example, you could have your first meal at 10am and finish eating by 6pm.

Many people succeed with this method as it's flexible enough for you to still enjoy dining out, no food groups are excluded, and you still get to eat adequate amounts of food each day.

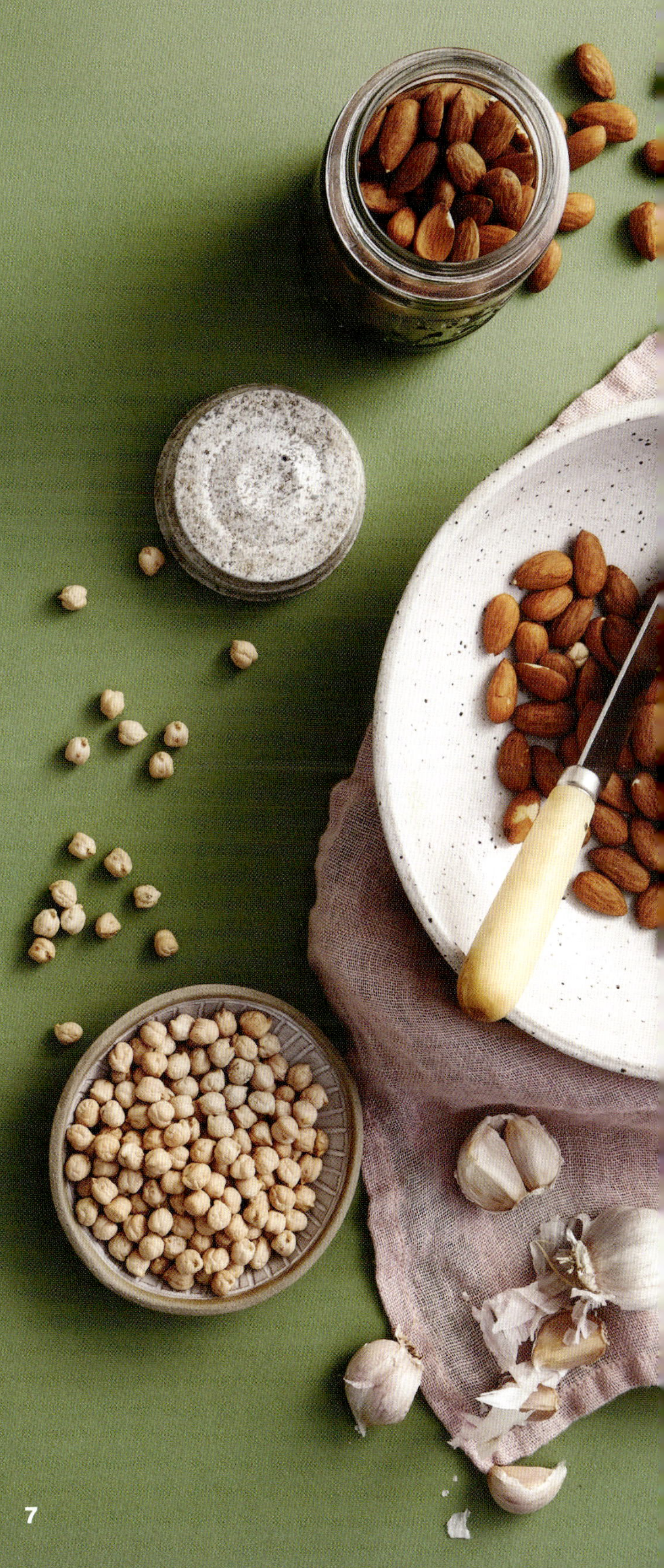

Intermittent fasting gives you **great flexibility** when choosing what to eat.

Intermittent fasting can be used without any food restrictions during your non-fasting window, or in conjunction with other dietary changes.

Essentially, you get to reap the benefits of fasting without going hungry or missing out!

WHAT TYPES OF FOOD SHOULD I BE EATING?

Intermittent fasting gives you great flexibility when choosing what to eat. No foods are completely off the table, but our bodies need a mix of protein, fats and carbohydrates to look after our health and wellbeing.

Despite what many other diet plans and philosophies say, no one food group is the problem. It's how much, when, and what types we choose to eat that can be problematic. Many of us tend to overdo it on carbohydrates, especially refined, processed ones such as cake, cookies, chips, white flour-based products and sugars.

When we eat, especially carbohydrate foods, our blood sugar levels rise, and the hormone insulin is released from the bloodstream, acting like a 'key' to unlock our cells to receive the energy from the food we've just eaten.

Any excess energy is stored in our fat cells for later use. If we are constantly eating, this process continues, and there is very little time for our body to lower our insulin levels and repair.

DO I NEED TO COUNT KILOJOULES?

When you're intermittent fasting, you don't need to count your energy intake (calories or kilojoules). By consuming your food within a shorter time frame, you'll often find yourself naturally eating less than usual.

However, it's important to consume enough kilojoules for your body to function and perform your daily tasks. This is not a starvation diet!

The average Australian adult tends to consume around 8700 kilojoules per day. Although, your individual needs vary significantly depending on your daily activity levels, age, sex, weight, height, and overall health status. For most men this sits around 10,700 kilojoules per day, while the average adult woman should aim to consume around 8,600 kilojoules per day.

The key to getting the most out of intermittent fasting is to make sure you're focusing on choosing quality food to promote good health.

We've compiled a variety of nourishing meals in this book to help you meet your nutritional needs so you can enjoy a wide variety of foods, improve your health, reach a healthy weight and forget kilojoule counting completely!

> *Despite what many other diet plans and philosophies may say, no one food group is the problem. It's how much, when, and what types we choose to eat that can be problematic.*

LIGHT MEALS

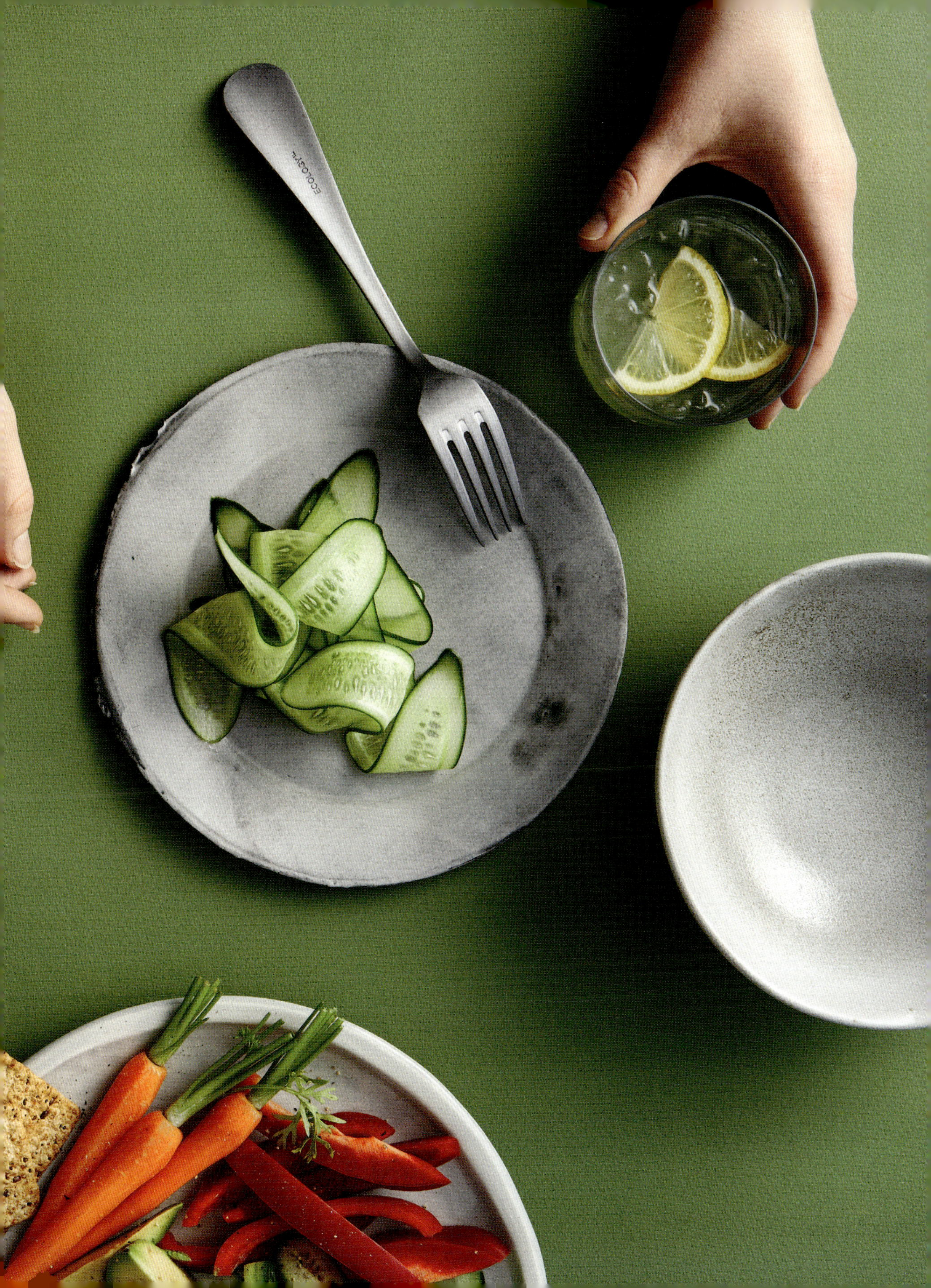
ECOLOGY™

PISTACHIO, CARDAMOM & ROSE QUINOA PORRIDGE

PREP + COOK TIME *20 MINUTES*
SERVES *2*

- **½ cup (100g) white quinoa, rinsed well**
- **1 cup (250ml) milk**
- **1 tsp ground cardamom**
- **½ tsp rosewater**
- **⅔ cup (190g) low-fat natural Greek yoghurt**
- **¼ cup (35g) coarsely chopped pistachios**
- **2 tsp dried food-grade rose petals, optional**
- **3 tsp maple syrup**

1 Place quinoa, milk, ½ cup (125ml) water, cardamom and rosewater in a medium heavy-based saucepan over medium heat; bring to the boil. Reduce heat to low; cook, stirring occasionally, for 15 minutes or until quinoa is softened and liquid absorbed.

2 Divide porridge between two bowls; top evenly with yoghurt, pistachios and rose petals. Drizzle with maple syrup to serve.

TIP If you don't have rosewater add vanilla extract or ½ teaspoon finely grated orange rind instead.

PREP IT If making ahead of time, add a little extra water to loosen up the quinoa porridge when reheating, as it will thicken on standing.

NUTRITION PER SERVING *15.9G TOTAL FAT (5G SATURATED FAT); 1430KJ (342 CAL); 31.6G CARBOHYDRATE; 15.9G PROTEIN; 4.5G FIBRE*

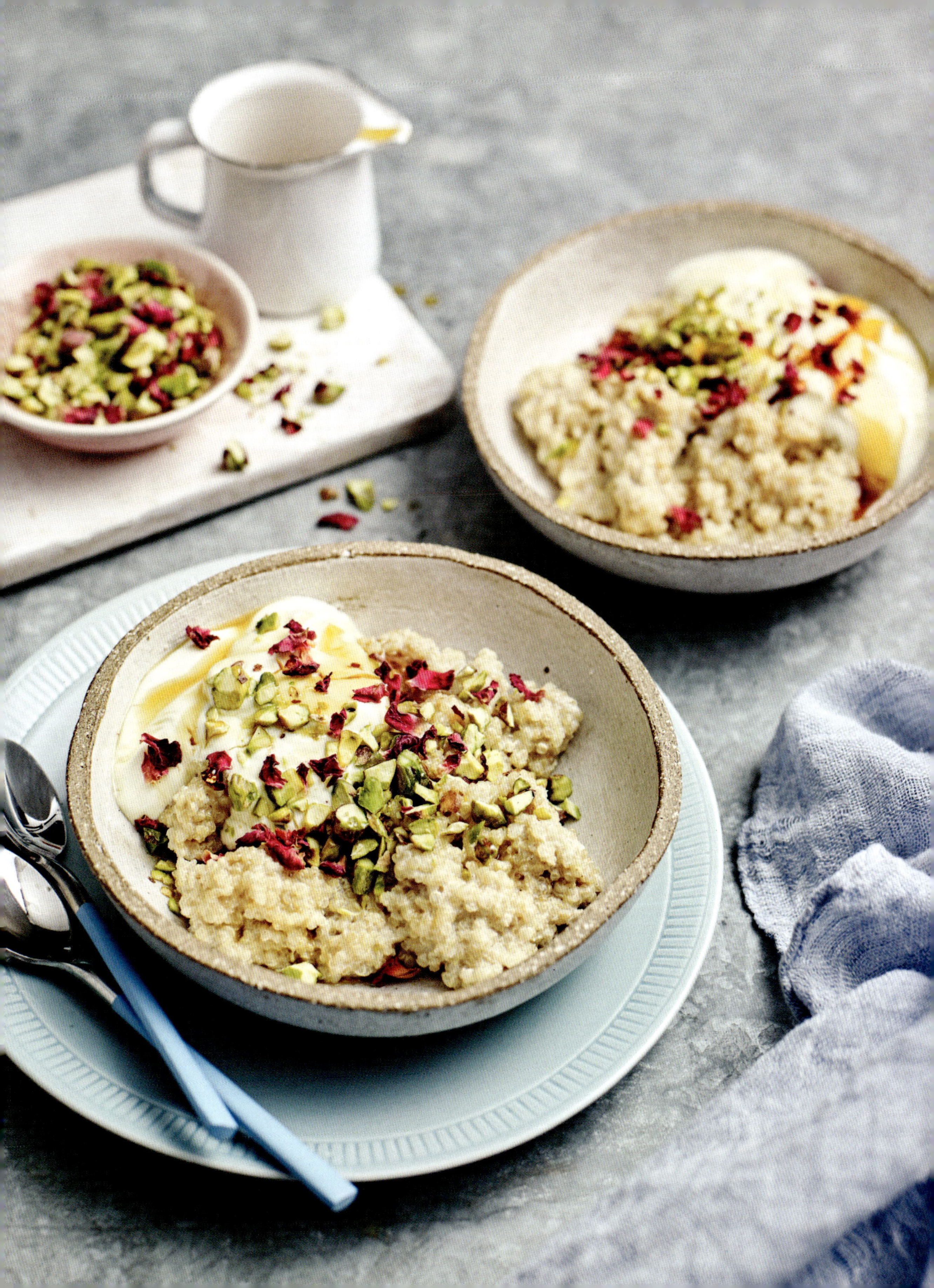

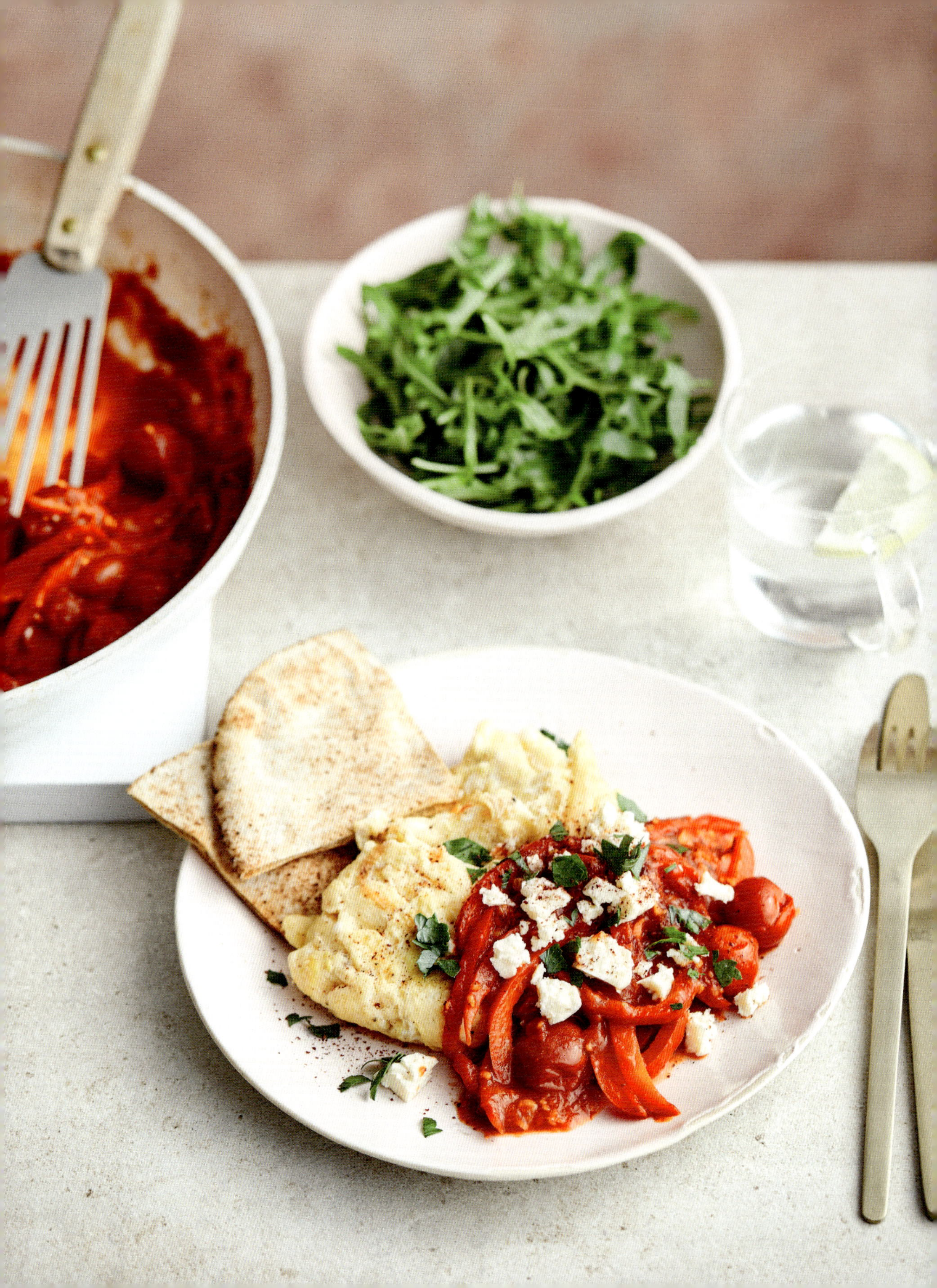

SCRAMBLED EGGS WITH CAPSICUM, FETTA & SUMAC

PREP + COOK TIME *15 MINUTES*
SERVES *2*

1 tsp extra virgin olive oil
4 green onions, chopped finely
1 medium red capsicum (200g), seeded, sliced thinly
400g can cherry tomatoes
3 extra-large eggs (60g each)
2 extra-large egg whites (from 60g eggs)
¼ cup (60ml) skim milk
extra virgin olive oil spray
1 wholemeal pitta bread pocket (50g), quartered
½ tsp ground sumac
30g reduced-fat fetta
⅓ cup coarsely chopped flat-leaf parsley
60g baby rocket leaves

1 Heat oil in a small frying pan over medium heat. Add green onion and capsicum; cook, stirring, for 5 minutes or until capsicum is soft. Add tomatoes; cook for a further 5 minutes or until slightly thickened. Season. Keep warm.

2 Meanwhile, whisk whole eggs, egg whites and milk in a medium bowl until combined; season. Spray a non-stick frying pan with a little oil spray, heat over medium-low heat. Add egg mixture; cook, stirring, for 3 minutes or until soft set.

3 Toast pitta bread. Sprinkle eggs with sumac and top with tomato mixture, crumbled fetta and parsley. Serve with toasted pitta and rocket.

NUTRITION PER SERVING *13.7G TOTAL FAT (4G SATURATED FAT); 1403KJ (335 CAL); 23.3G CARBOHYDRATE; 25.7G PROTEIN; 6.9G FIBRE*

BANANA & COCONUT PORRIDGE

PREP + COOK TIME *20 MINUTES*
SERVES 4

- **400ml can coconut milk**
- **4 medium bananas (800g)**
- **4 makrut lime leaves**
- **2 cups (180g) rolled oats**
- **1 tsp finely grated lime rind**
- **2 tsp lime juice**
- **1 tbsp rice malt syrup**
- **½ cup (35g) coconut flakes, toasted**

1 Reserve 2 tablespoons of the coconut milk to serve. Break 2 bananas into pieces; tear 2 lime leaves. Place banana pieces and torn lime leaves into a blender or food processor with remaining coconut milk; blend until smooth.

2 Pour banana mixture into a large saucepan, then add oats and 2 cups (500ml) water. Bring to a simmer over medium heat. Reduce heat to low; cook, stirring frequently, for 7 minutes or until oats are tender.

3 Meanwhile, cut the centre vein from remaining lime leaves and discard; stack leaves, then shred very finely. Slice remaining bananas.

4 Stir lime rind, lime juice and rice malt syrup through porridge; spoon into bowls. Serve topped with reserved coconut milk, the sliced banana, coconut flakes and shredded lime leaves.

TIP Leftover makrut lime leaves can be frozen for another use.

NUTRITION PER SERVING *22.9G TOTAL FAT (16.3G SATURATED FAT); 2358KJ (564 CAL); 74.1G CARBOHYDRATE; 9.3G PROTEIN; 10.4G FIBRE*

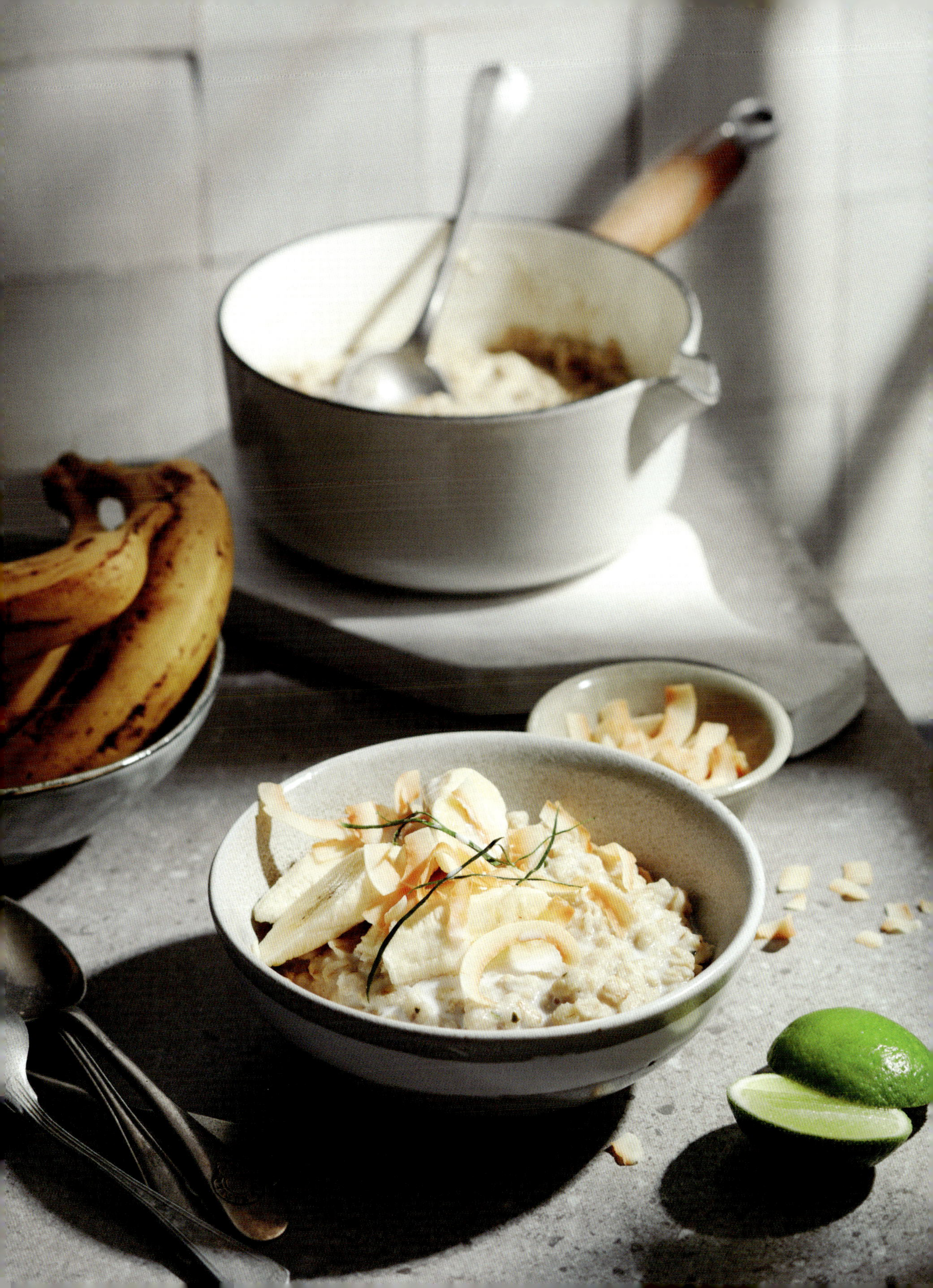

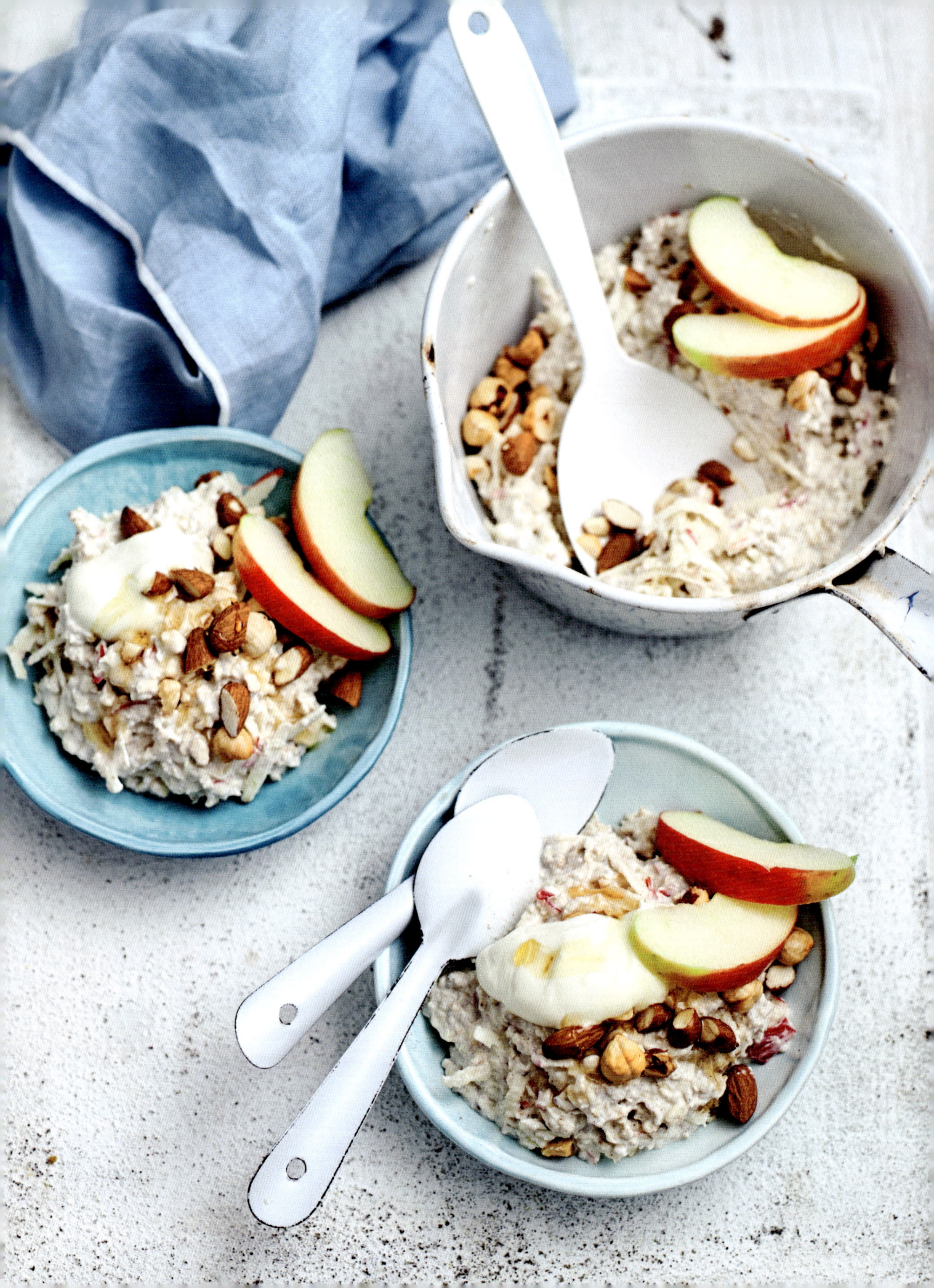

CHIA & APPLE OAT BIRCHER

PREP + COOK TIME *10 MINUTES (+ STANDING)*
SERVES *4*

- **1⅓ cups (375g) Greek yoghurt**
- **1 cup (250ml) milk**
- **1 tbsp chia seeds**
- **1½ cups (135g) rolled oats**
- **2 medium red apples (300g)**
- **½ tsp ground cinnamon**
- **¼ tsp ground cardamom**
- **⅓ cup (45g) chopped roasted hazelnuts**
- **¼ cup (40g) chopped roasted natural almonds**
- **1 tbsp honey**

1 Combine 1 cup of the yoghurt, the milk, chia seeds and oats in a medium bowl. Stand for 15 minutes.

2 Meanwhile, coarsely grate 1½ apples. Add grated apple and the spices to oat mixture; stir to mix well.

3 Cut remaining apple into eight thin wedges. Divide oat mixture evenly among four bowls; top with remaining yoghurt and apple slices. Sprinkle with combined chopped nuts and drizzle with honey to serve.

PREP IT Divide bircher into 4 portions at the end of step 2. Refrigerate for up to 4 days. To serve, top each portion with 1 tablespoon yoghurt and 2 pieces of sliced apple. Sprinkle with combined chopped nuts and drizzle with honey.

NUTRITION PER SERVING *22.4G TOTAL FAT (4.7G SATURATED FAT); 2005KJ (479 CAL); 50.7G CARBOHYDRATE; 15G PROTEIN; 7.7G FIBRE*

BIG MUSHROOMS WITH FETTA & SPINACH

PREP + COOK TIME *30 MINUTES*
SERVES 4

4 portobello mushrooms (200g)
2 tbsp extra virgin olive oil
1 eschalot, chopped finely
½ tsp ground nutmeg
200g baby spinach leaves
4 slices soy and linseed bread (280g)
1 clove garlic, peeled, halved
100g reduced-fat fetta, crumbled
2 tbsp pepitas (pumpkin seed kernels), toasted

1 Preheat oven to 200°C. Line a large oven tray with baking paper.

2 Place mushrooms on tray; bake for 15 minutes or until browned and softened slightly.

3 Meanwhile, heat 1 tablespoon of the oil in a medium frying pan over medium heat. Cook eschalot, stirring, for 4 minutes or until light golden. Add nutmeg; stir to combine. Add spinach and 1 tablespoon water; cook, stirring, for 1 minute or until just wilted. Stir in any mushroom juices left on the oven tray.

4 Heat a grill plate (or grill pan) over medium-high heat; grill bread for 2 minutes each side or until toasted and grill marks appear. Rub cut side of garlic clove over one side of each piece of toast.

5 Top each mushroom evenly with spinach mixture; sprinkle evenly with fetta and pepitas. Drizzle with remaining oil; serve with toast.

TIP Instead of chargrilling the bread, you can toast in a toaster, if preferred.

NUTRITION PER SERVING *20.1G TOTAL FAT (4.6G SATURATED FAT); 1522KJ (363 CAL); 24.2G CARBOHYDRATE; 17.1G PROTEIN; 7.7G FIBRE*

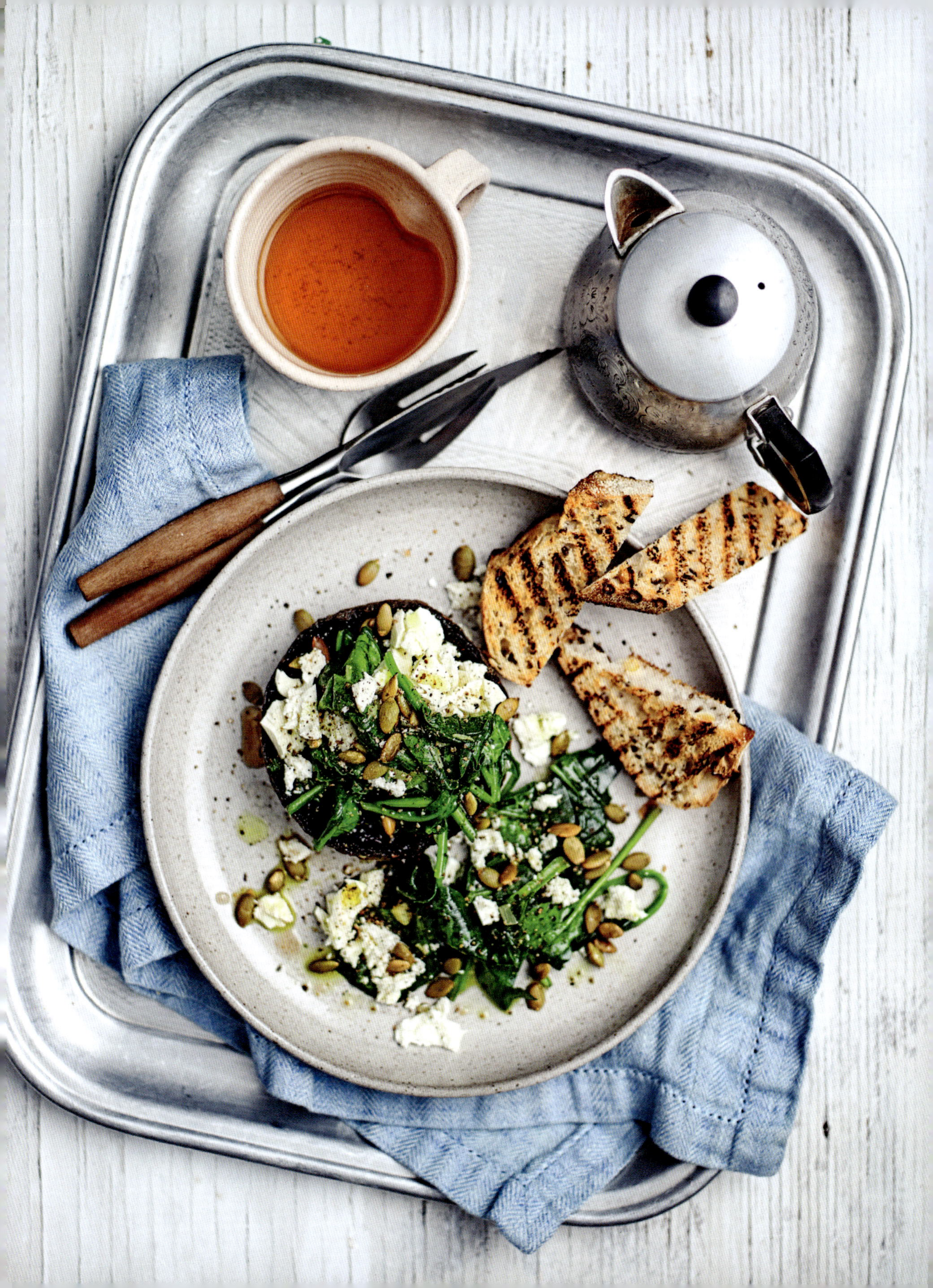

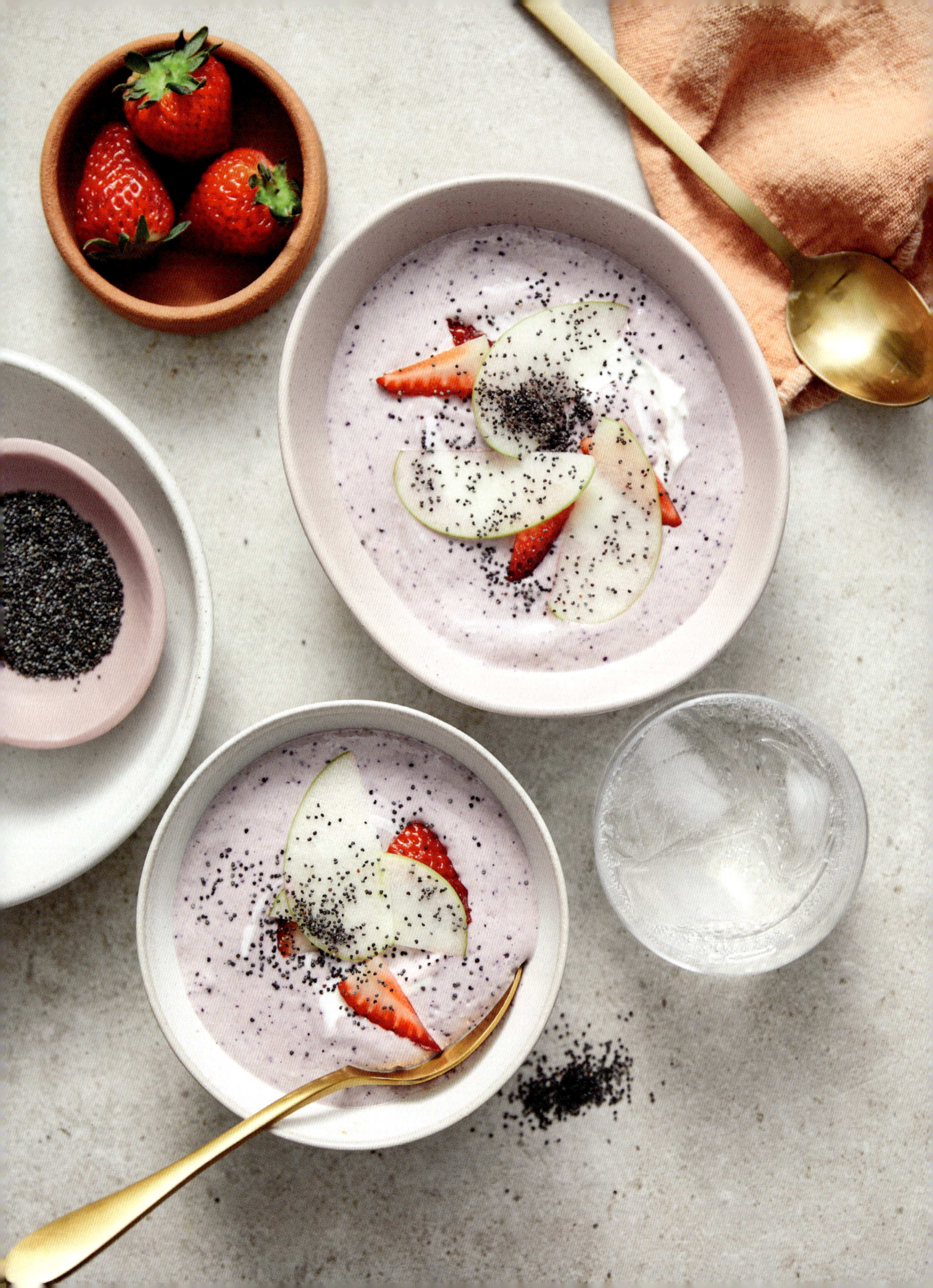

TOFU & BERRY BREAKFAST SMOOTHIE BOWL

PREP TIME *5 MINUTES*
SERVES *2*

100g rolled oats
150g silken tofu
⅓ cup (50g) blueberries
1 tsp vanilla bean paste
1 tsp maple syrup
1 cup (250ml) ice cubes
1 medium green apple (150g), cored, sliced thinly
1½ cups (195g) strawberries, trimmed, halved
¾ cup (200g) high-protein natural yoghurt
½ tsp poppy seeds

1 Blend oats, tofu, blueberries, vanilla, maple syrup and ice cubes with half the apple, strawberries and yoghurt in a high-powered blender until very smooth.

2 Pour smoothie evenly between two bowls, top with remaining apple slices, strawberries and yoghurt; sprinkle with poppy seeds.

TIP You could also use raspberries or blackberries instead of the strawberries and blueberries in this recipe, if preferred.

NUTRITION PER SERVING *6.5G TOTAL FAT (1.1G SATURATED FAT); 1536KJ (367 CAL); 47.2G CARBOHYDRATE; 22.6G PROTEIN; 14G FIBRE*

BLUEBERRY PIE JAR

PREP TIME *25 MINUTES (+ STANDING)*
SERVES *4*

250g blueberries

2 medium yellow peaches (300g), cut into 2cm pieces

1 medium apple (150g), cut into 2cm pieces

1 tsp ground cinnamon

1 tsp vanilla bean paste

1 tsp finely grated lemon rind

⅓ cup (80ml) maple syrup

3 cups (360g) almond hazelnut granola (see tip)

2 cups (560g) Greek yoghurt

1 Place blueberries, peaches, apple, cinnamon, vanilla, lemon rind and 2 tablespoons maple syrup in a medium bowl; stir to combine. Cover; stand for 30 minutes.

2 Meanwhile, process granola until coarsely chopped. Add remaining maple syrup; pulse until just combined.

3 Divide fruit mixture among four 1½-cup (375ml) jars; top with granola mixture. Serve with yoghurt.

TIP You can use your favourite granola for this recipe, if you like.

NUTRITION PER SERVING *19.5G TOTAL FAT (5.2G SATURATED FAT); 2948KJ (705 CAL); 103.3G CARBOHYDRATE; 22.3G PROTEIN; 12.2G FIBRE*

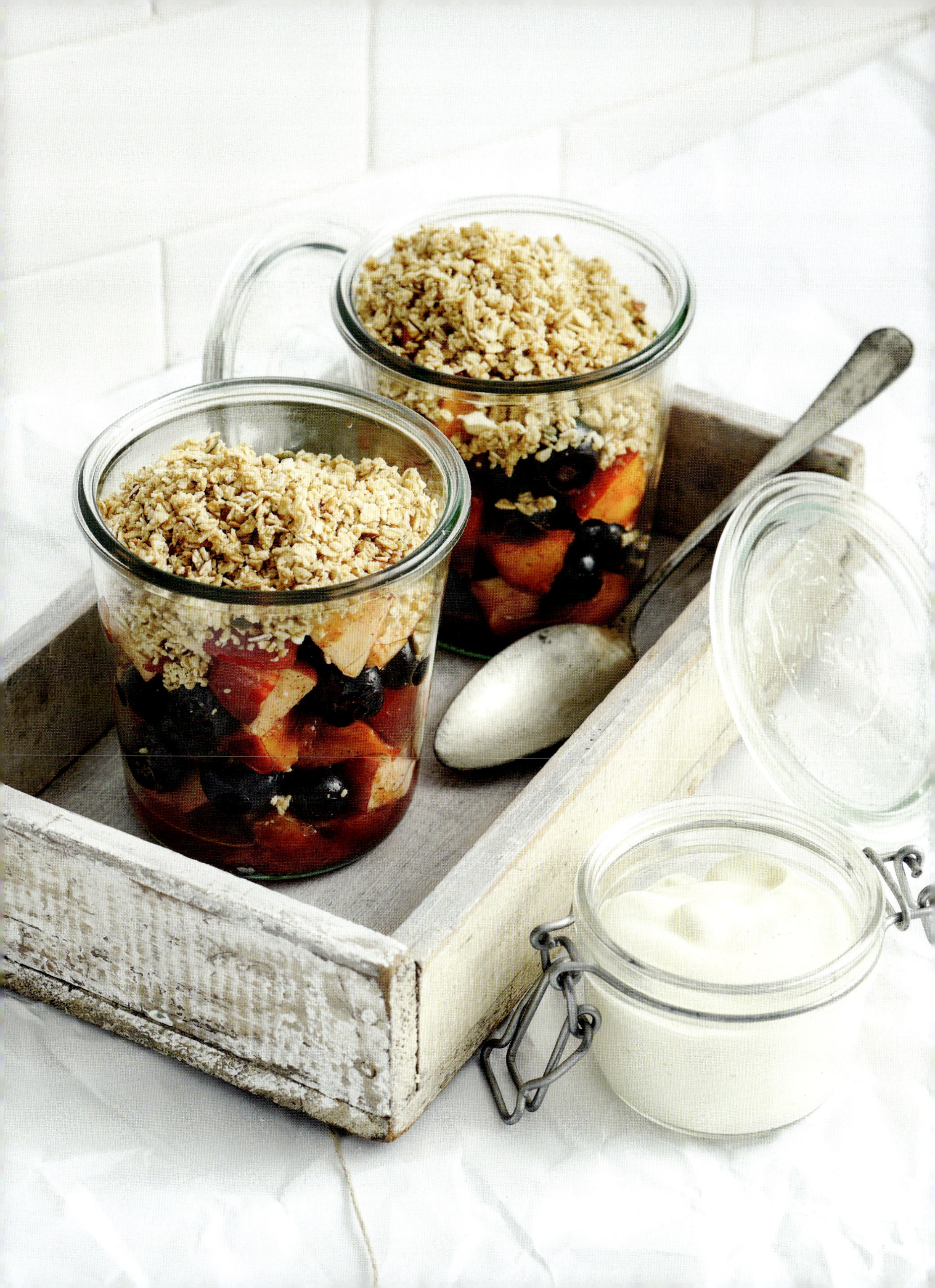

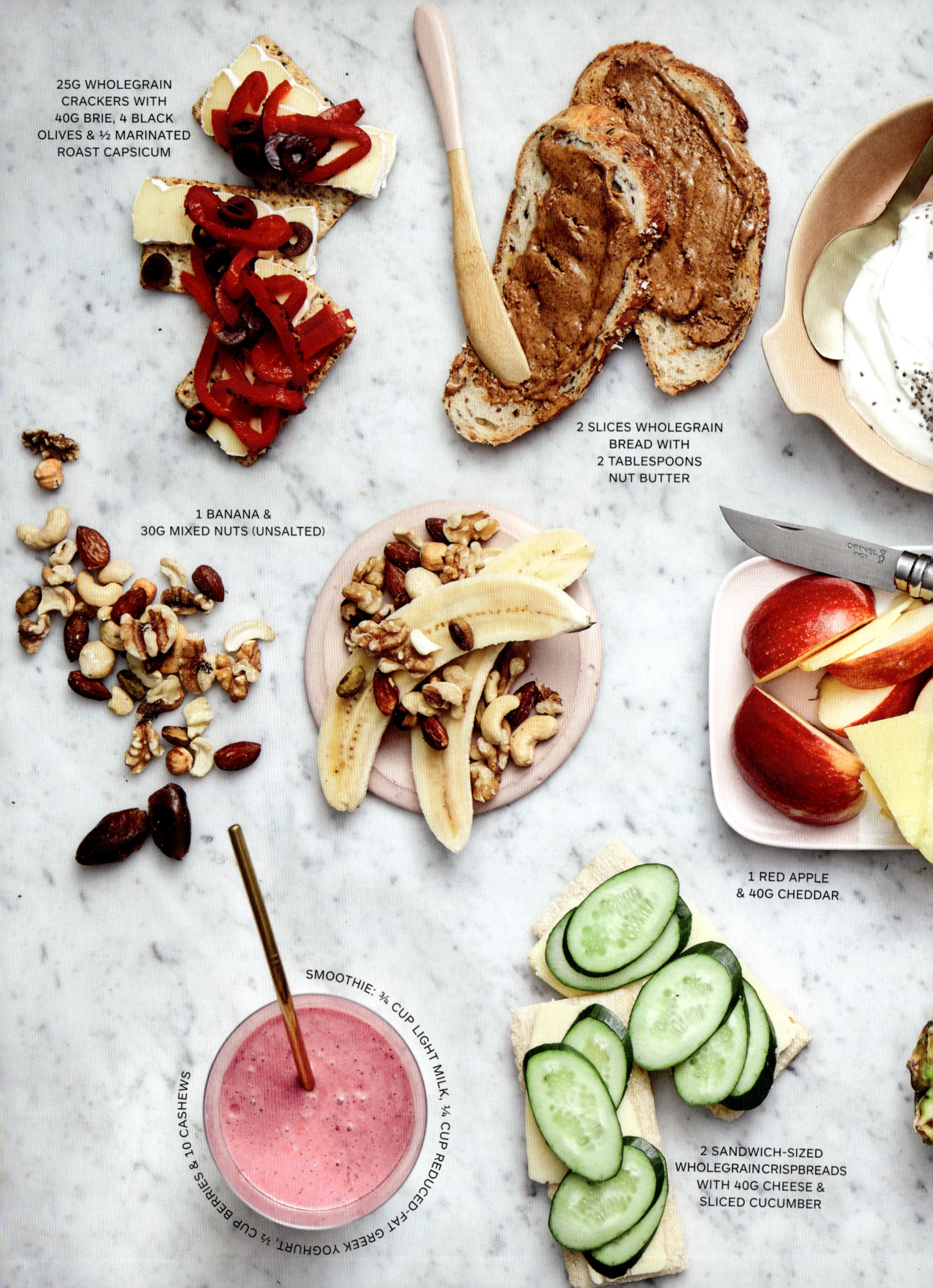
25G WHOLEGRAIN CRACKERS WITH 40G BRIE, 4 BLACK OLIVES & ½ MARINATED ROAST CAPSICUM
2 SLICES WHOLEGRAIN BREAD WITH 2 TABLESPOONS NUT BUTTER
1 BANANA & 30G MIXED NUTS (UNSALTED)
1 RED APPLE & 40G CHEDDAR
SMOOTHIE: ¾ CUP LIGHT MILK, ¼ CUP REDUCED-FAT GREEK YOGHURT, ½ CUP BERRIES & 10 CASHEWS
2 SANDWICH-SIZED WHOLEGRAINCRISPBREADS WITH 40G CHEESE & SLICED CUCUMBER

SNACK IDEAS

SWEET + SAVOURY

½ CUP MIXED BERRIES, 200G REDUCED-FAT GREEK YOGHURT & ½ TABLESPOON CHIA SEEDS (OR 10 ALMONDS)
20G AIR-POPPED PLAIN POPCORN & 1 BANANA
2 WHOLEGRAIN CRACKERS WITH ½ AVOCADO & 1 SLICED TOMATO
¼ CUP HUMMUS WITH 1 CARROT & A CELERY STICK, CUT INTO BATONS
1 CUP CHOPPED PINEAPPLE

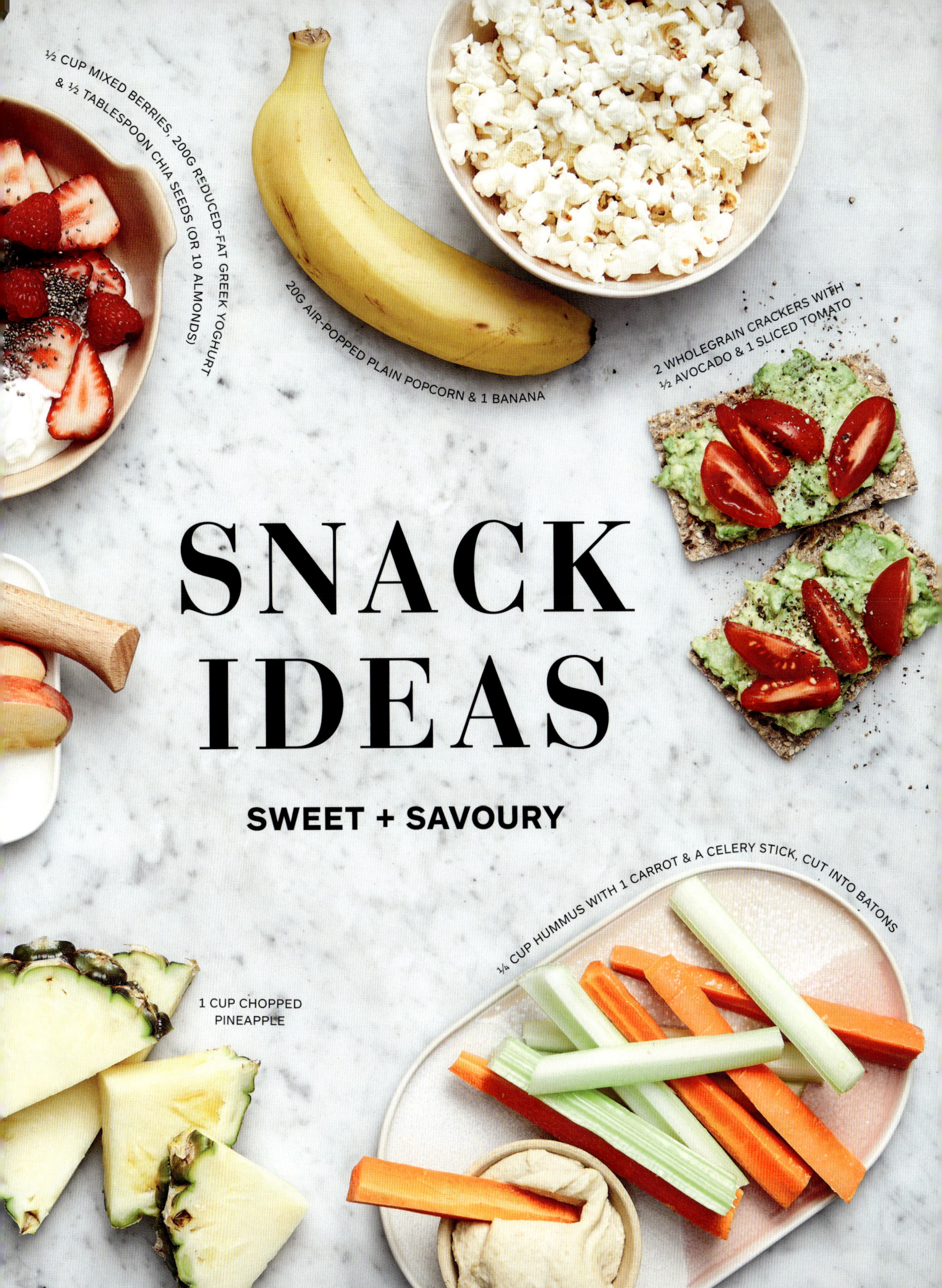

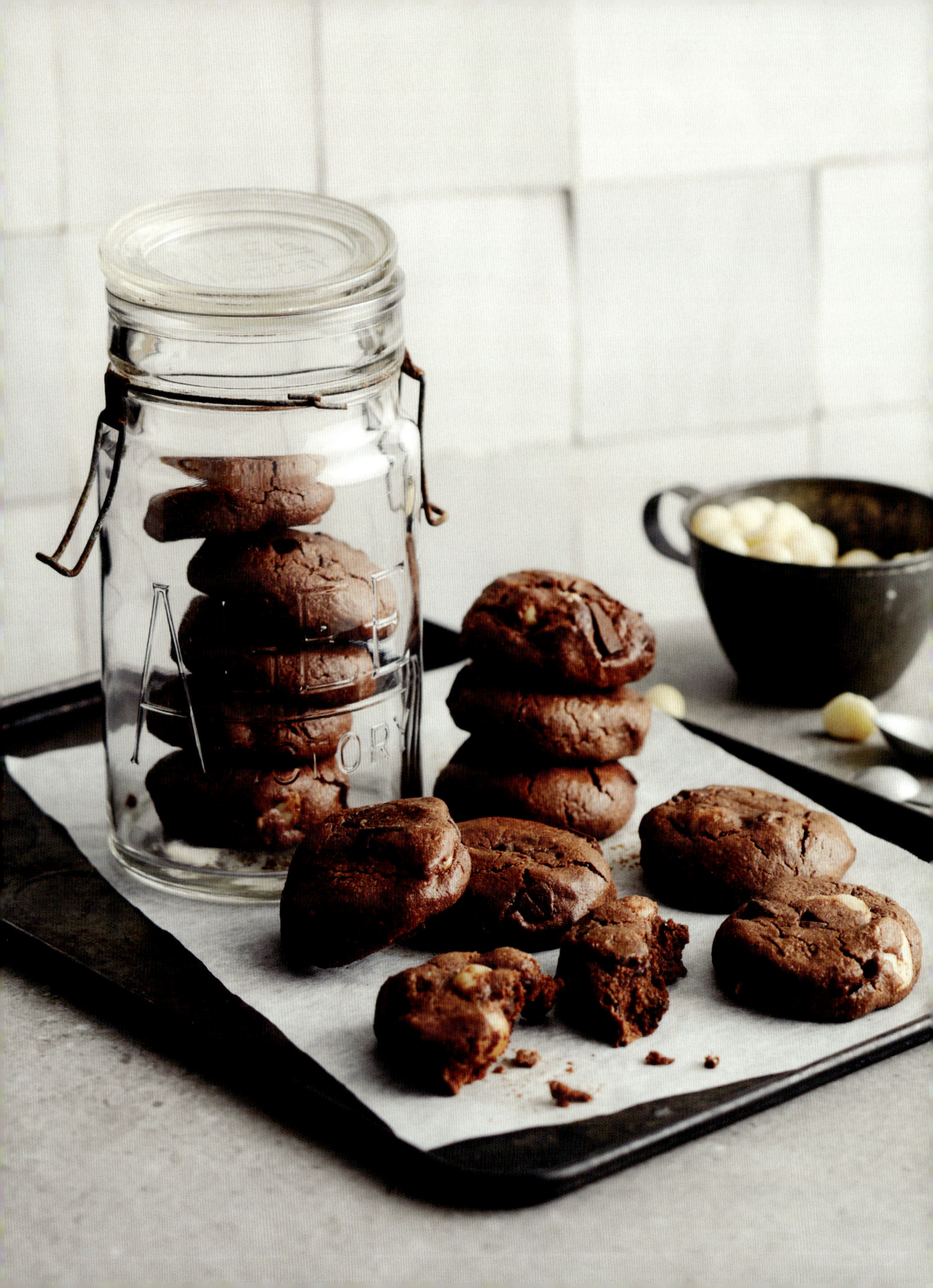

CHOC-GINGER COOKIES

PREP + COOK TIME *25 MINUTES*
MAKES *12*

1¼ cups (150g) almond meal

¼ cup (25g) cacao powder

1½ tsp ground ginger

1 tsp ground cinnamon

½ tsp gluten-free baking powder

¼ cup (60ml) extra virgin olive oil

¼ cup (60ml) maple syrup

1 tbsp almond butter

1 egg

1 tsp vanilla extract

80g dark chocolate (85% cocoa), broken into 1cm pieces

½ cup (70g) unsalted macadamias, halved

1 Preheat oven to 180°C. Line a large oven tray with baking paper.

2 Combine almond meal, cacao powder, ginger, cinnamon and baking powder in a medium bowl.

3 In another bowl, whisk oil, maple syrup, almond butter, egg and vanilla until well combined and smooth. Add wet mixture to dry ingredients; stir until just combined. Gently stir in chocolate and macadamias. Stand mixture for 5 minutes to firm up a little.

4 Using damp hands, roll 1½ tablespoons of the mixture into balls, place on trays; flatten with the palm of your hand into 5cm rounds.

5 Bake for 10 minutes or until cookies can be gently pushed without breaking. Cool on tray.

TIP Store cookies in an airtight container at room temperature for up to 3 days.

NUTRITION PER COOKIE *19.8G TOTAL FAT (3.7G SATURATED FAT); 998KJ (239 CAL); 10.1G CARBOHYDRATE; 4.8G PROTEIN; 2.4G FIBRE*

BANANA OAT MUFFINS

PREP + COOK TIME *40 MINUTES (+ COOLING)*
MAKES 6

- **cooking oil spray**
- **1½ cups (135g) rolled oats**
- **½ cup (80g) wholemeal plain (all-purpose) flour**
- **1 tsp ground nutmeg**
- **½ tsp bicarbonate of soda (baking soda)**
- **1 tsp baking powder**
- **½ cup (55g) coarsely chopped walnuts**
- **120g apple sauce**
- **2 extra-large eggs (60g each), beaten lightly**
- **¼ cup (60ml) milk**
- **½ cup (140g) Greek yoghurt**
- **¾ cup (210g) mashed ripe banana (see tip)**
- **1½ tbsp honey**
- **1 medium banana (200g), extra, cut into 12 slices**
- **2 tsp lemon juice**
- **⅔ cup (185g) Greek yoghurt, extra**

1 Preheat oven to 200°C. Lightly spray a 6-hole (¾-cup/180ml) Texas muffin pan with oil spray; line base and side with two overlapping strips of baking paper.

2 Reserve 1 tablespoon of the oats. Process remaining oats until chopped finely but still retaining some texture. Combine chopped oats, flour, nutmeg, bicarb, baking powder and half of the walnuts in a large bowl. Make a well in the centre; pour in combined apple sauce, egg, milk, yoghurt, mashed banana and 1 tablespoon of the honey. Stir until just combined, taking care not to over-mix. Spoon batter evenly into pan holes.

3 Combine sliced banana and lemon juice in a small bowl. Place 2 banana slices on each muffin; sprinkle evenly with the reserved oats and remaining walnuts.

4 Bake for 25 minutes or until muffins are golden and cooked when a skewer inserted into the centre comes out clean. Cool muffins in pan for 5 minutes before turning, top-side up, onto a wire rack to cool completely.

5 Top muffins with extra yoghurt. Drizzle with remaining honey just before serving.

TIP You will need to mash about 2 medium bananas for this recipe.

NUTRITION PER MUFFIN *16.3G TOTAL FAT (5G SATURATED FAT); 1633KJ (390 CAL); 46.6G CARBOHYDRATE; 11.4G PROTEIN; 5.9G FIBRE*

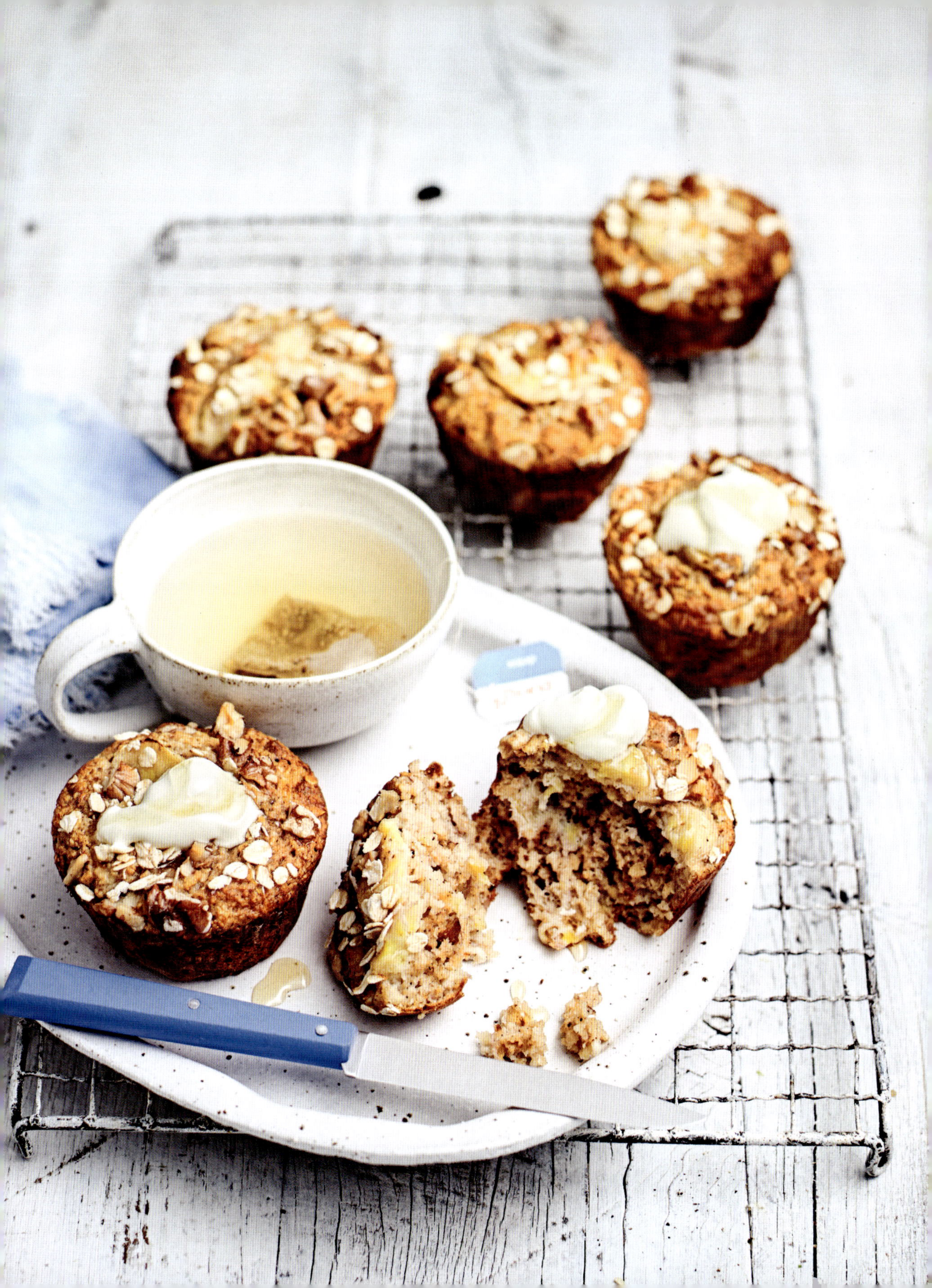

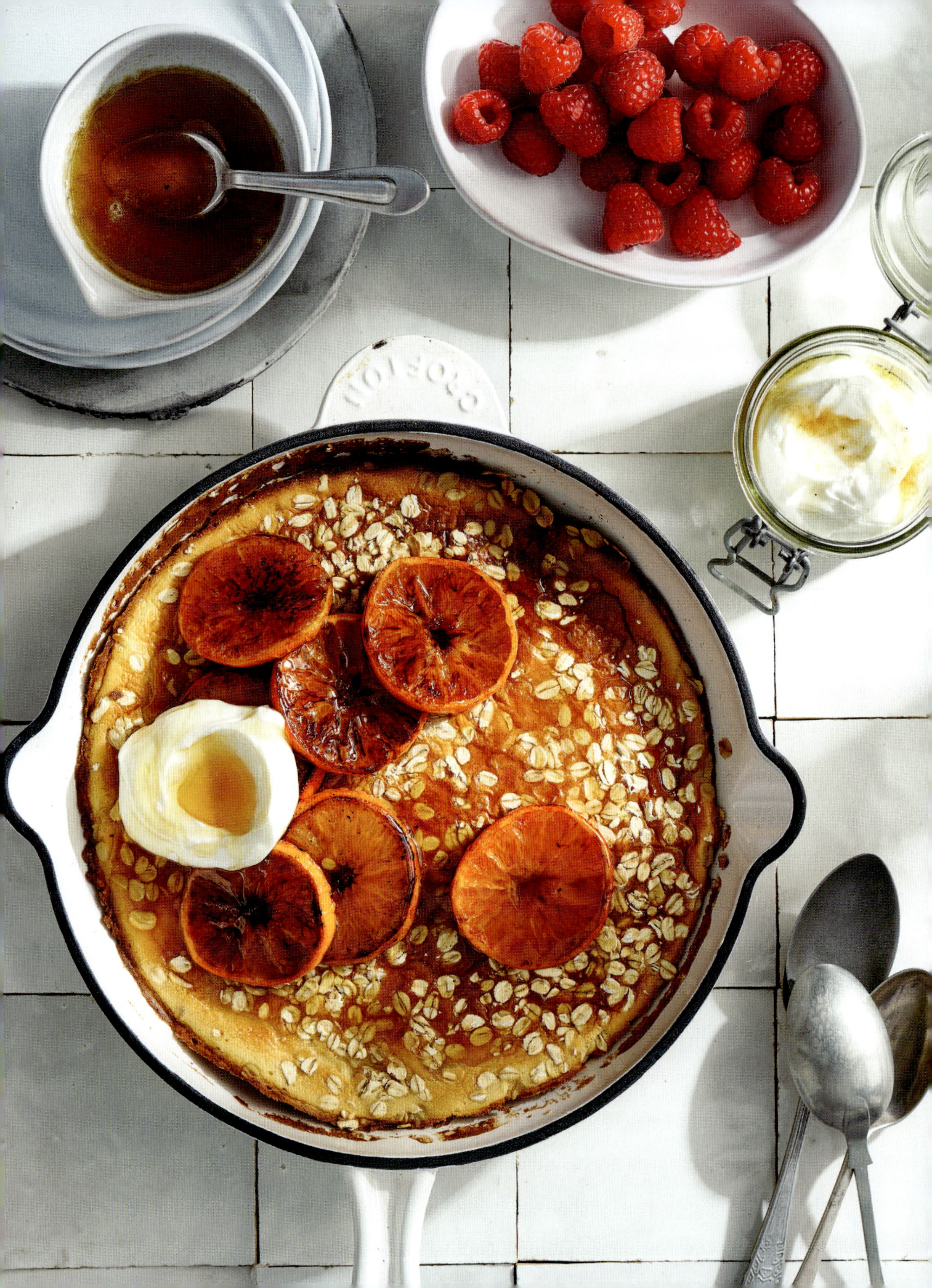
CROFTON

DUTCH PANCAKE WITH HONEY MANDARINS

PREP + COOK TIME *35 MINUTES*
SERVES *4*

3 extra-large eggs (60g each), at room temperature

¾ cup (105g) white spelt flour

pinch of salt

1 tsp baking powder

2 tbsp unrefined sugar (see tip)

1 cup (250ml) lukewarm milk

1 tsp vanilla bean paste

2 tbsp extra virgin olive oil

2 tbsp rolled oats

3 seedless mandarins (300g)

¼ cup (90g) honey

1 cup (280g) high-protein natural yoghurt

125g raspberries

1 Preheat oven to 220°C. Place a 26cm cast-iron pan or ovenproof frying pan in oven while heating until pan is very hot.

2 Meanwhile, blend eggs for 2 minutes or until frothy. Sift flour, salt, baking powder and sugar onto a piece of baking paper. With the motor operating, pour in combined milk and vanilla, then quickly add the sifted flour mixture. Blend for a further 10 seconds until just combined.

3 Working quickly, add 1 tablespoon of the olive oil to the hot pan, swirling to cover base. Pour batter into pan, then scatter with oats; immediately return pan to the oven. Bake for 20 minutes or until pancake is puffed and browned at the edge.

4 Meanwhile, cut unpeeled mandarins into 5mm thick slices. Heat remaining oil in a non-stick frying pan; cook mandarin slices, in two batches, for 1 minute each side or until lightly browned. Remove from pan. Add honey and ¼ cup (60ml) water; simmer for 1 minute. Return mandarin slices to pan; coat in syrup.

5 Top pancake with mandarin slices and yoghurt; drizzle with remaining syrup. Serve with raspberries.

TIP Use any type of unrefined sugar such as rapadura or panela.

NUTRITION PER SERVING *16.3G TOTAL FAT (4.1G SATURATED FAT); 2045KJ (489 CAL); 62.1G CARBOHYDRATE; 21.4G PROTEIN; 5.3G FIBRE*

CRUNCHY BANANA & VANILLA YOGHURT TOAST

PREP + COOK TIME *10 MINUTES*
SERVES 4

½ cup (140g) Greek yoghurt (see tip)

1 tsp vanilla bean paste

4 slices soy and linseed sourdough bread (280g)

2 medium bananas (400g), sliced

1 tsp linseeds (flaxseeds), toasted

2 tsp sunflower seeds, toasted

1 tsp black chia seeds, toasted

1 tbsp honey

1 Combine yoghurt and vanilla in a small bowl.

2 Toast bread; spread evenly with vanilla yoghurt. Top with banana slices and combined toasted seeds. Drizzle toast evenly with honey to serve.

TIP Choose a Greek yoghurt that doesn't contain added sugar.

NUTRITION PER SERVING *5.7G TOTAL FAT (1.5G SATURATED FAT); 1306KJ (312 CAL); 52.9G CARBOHYDRATE; 11.1G PROTEIN; 3.6G FIBRE*

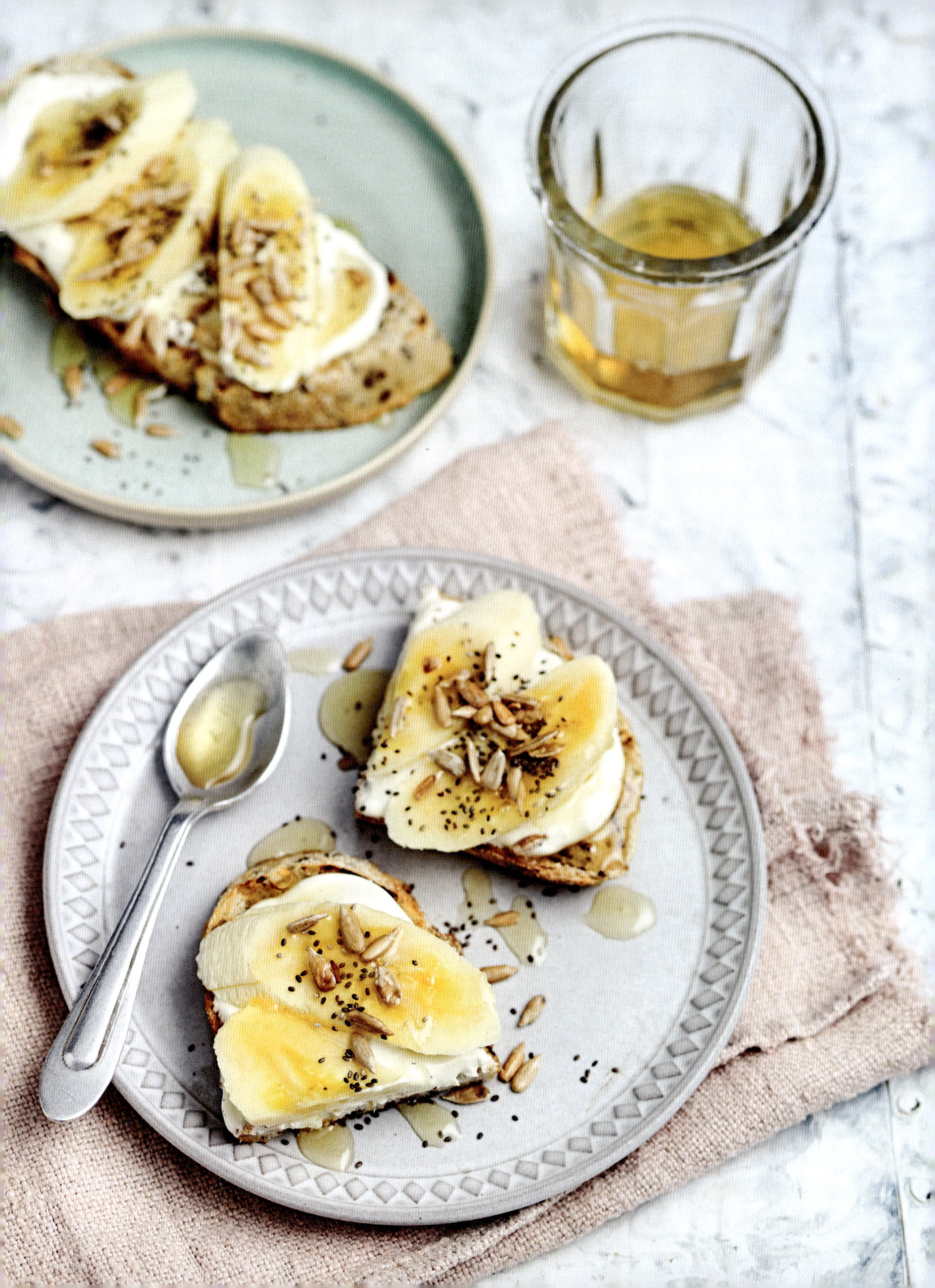

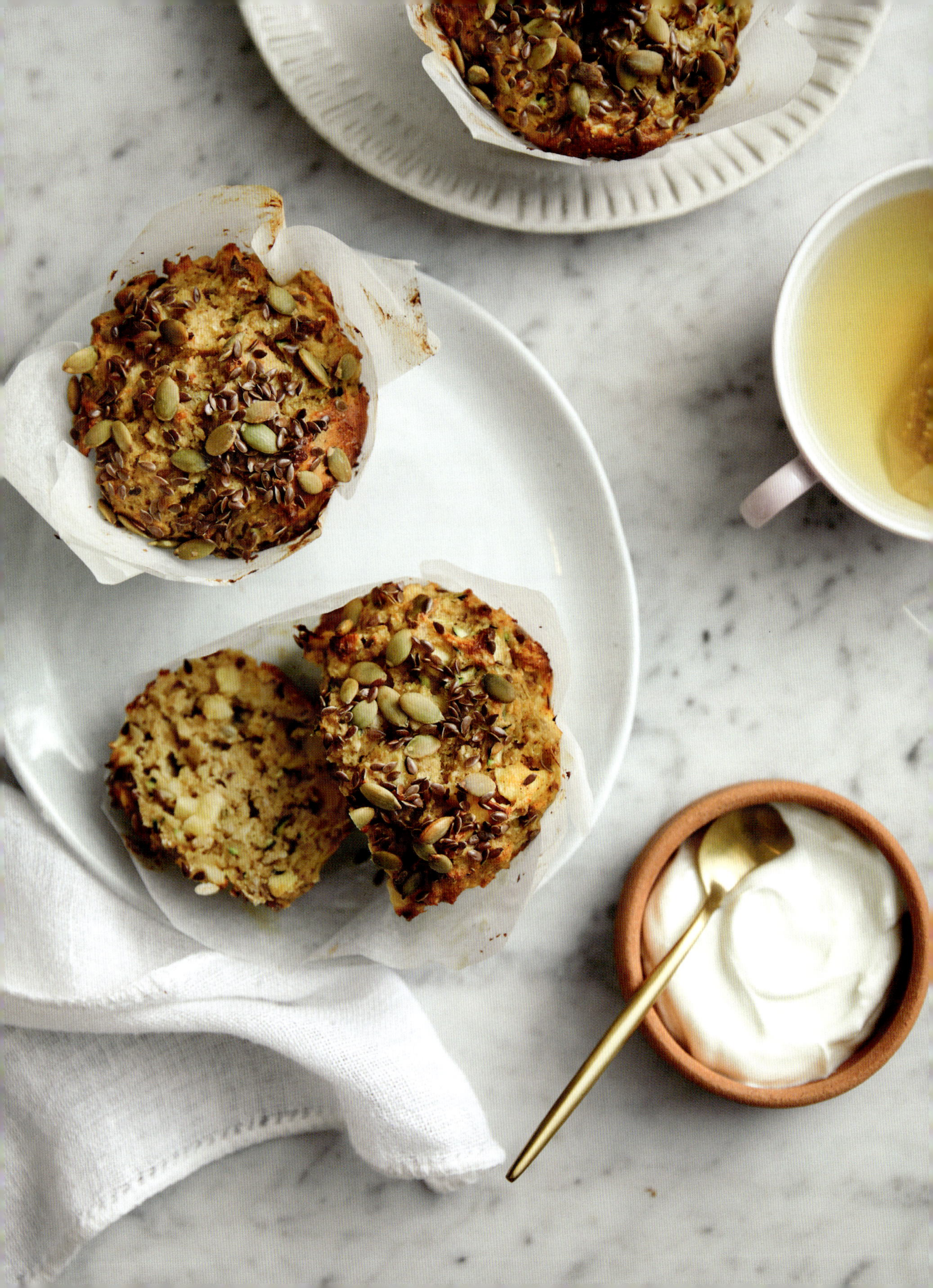

EARL GREY, APPLE & ZUCCHINI MUFFINS

PREP + COOK TIME *40 MINUTES (+ STANDING)*
MAKES *4*

- **1 earl grey tea bag**
- **80g dried apples, chopped into 5mm pieces**
- **½ cup (45g) rolled oats**
- **1 medium zucchini (120g), grated, squeezed lightly**
- **1½ cups (420g) high-protein natural yoghurt**
- **1 egg**
- **2 tsp maple syrup**
- **½ cup (80g) wholemeal self-raising flour**
- **½ cup (50g) lupin flour (see tips)**
- **1¼ tsp baking powder**
- **1 tsp ground ginger**
- **1 tsp mixed spice**
- **1 tbsp linseeds (flaxseeds)**
- **1 tbsp pepitas (pumpkin seed kernels)**

1 Preheat oven to 200°C. Line 4 holes of a ¾-cup (180ml) Texas muffin pan with non-stick cafe-style muffin cases or squares of baking paper.

2 Place tea bag in 1 cup (250ml) boiling water for 5 minutes. Place apples, oats and brewed tea in a medium bowl; mix well. Stand for 20 minutes or until most of the liquid is absorbed. Stir in zucchini, ½ cup (140g) of the yoghurt, the egg and maple syrup.

3 Sift flours, baking powder and spices into a large bowl; return husks to the bowl. Make a well in the centre; stir in zucchini mixture with half each of the linseeds and pepitas. Mixture will be quite thick. Spoon mixture evenly into paper cases, sprinkle with remaining linseeds and pepitas.

4 Bake muffins for 30 minutes or until a skewer inserted in the centre of a muffin comes out clean. If muffins start to overbrown, cover loosely with foil. Stand for 5 minutes before placing on a wire rack to cool. Serve muffins warm with remaining yoghurt.

TIPS Lupin flour is made by processing whole dried lupin beans into flour. They are a protein and fibre-rich legume (belonging to the same family as beans, peas, lentils and peanuts), and are gluten free. They are also low in carbohydrates and have a low GI. Lupin flour is available from major supermarkets and health food stores. Muffins are best eaten on day of baking and can be frozen for up to 1 month.

NUTRITION PER MUFFIN *6.7G TOTAL FAT (1.2G SATURATED FAT); 1377KJ (328 CAL); 41G CARBOHYDRATE; 22.3G PROTEIN; 11.2G FIBRE*

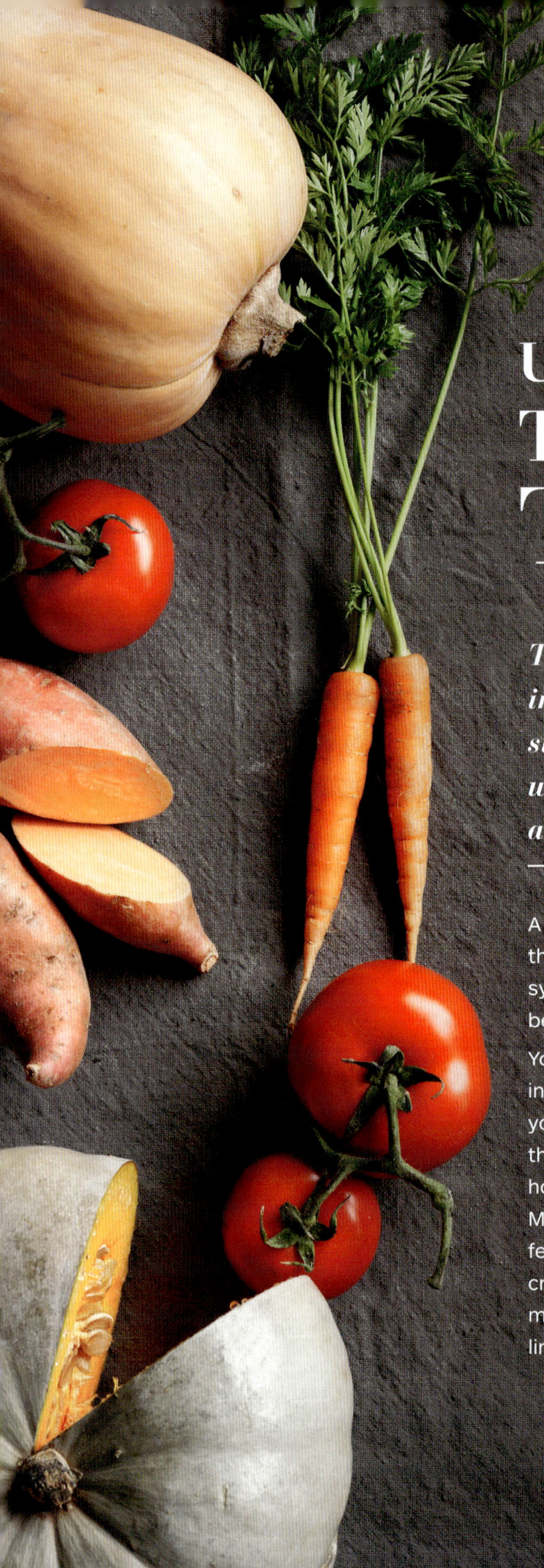

UNDERSTANDING THE ROLE OF THE GUT

There are trillions of bacteria in your body, some of which support good health, and others which can have negative effects and contribute to disease.

A diet rich in prebiotic foods helps to feed the beneficial gut bacteria in our digestive system, which results in a whole host of beneficial outcomes for our bodies.

Your gut bacteria play a significant role in how you digest certain foods and how you store fat. They also produce chemicals that help you to feel full, and influence the hormones that regulate your appetite. Mood swings, sugar cravings and constantly feeling under the weather? These little critters also play a role in regulating your mood and blood sugar, and form the first line of defence for your immune system.

HOW HEALTHY IS YOUR GUT?

When determining what to eat, many of us only think about how quick the food is to prepare, and will it taste good? Your gut, on the other hand, has other needs that, when met, supports overall health and our weight-loss efforts.

Gut health and weight loss is a relatively new research area, yet scientists can already predict if a person is overweight or lean by a sample of their gut bacteria.

Certain gut microbes seem to play a role in obesity with new weight-loss research targeting the gut microbiota to determine which strains of bacteria have the biggest impact. So far, it seems that slimmer people tend to have 70% more gut bacteria as well as a more diverse microbiome than their overweight peers.

HOW YOUR GUT HEALTH AFFECTS YOUR WEIGHT

There appears to be three key ways an imbalance in your gut bacteria could be making it hard for you to lose weight. This includes chronic inflammation, a lack of butyrate production, and your bacteria's influence on the hormones that make you feel hungry. Some evidence suggests chronic inflammation can contribute to obesity by leading to increased fat storage. When you have an imbalance of gut bacteria, certain problematic microbes can add to this overall body inflammation by producing by-products that enter the bloodstream and turn on your body's inflammatory responses.

In contract, healthy bacteria produce short-chain fatty acids, such as butyrate, that improve health. This important short-chain fatty acid is protective against obesity and insulin resistance, a precursor to Type 2 diabetes. Butyrate also reduces overall body inflammation, and makes you feel full quicker.

Thirdly, certain microbes influence the hormones that control our hunger and satiety. Current research suggests you'll feel hungrier if you have a low diversity of gut bacteria, especially if they aren't producing enough enzymes or butyrate.

IMPROVING YOUR GUT HEALTH WITH FOOD

It's important to talk with your doctor first, but if you're experiencing heartburn, excessive fullness, excessive burping, nausea, rumbling stomach noises, bloating, abdominal pain, abnormal bowel habits, and excessive wind, these can all be signs of an unhappy gut. A diet with plenty of fibre from a diverse range of whole foods, probiotic-rich foods including yoghurt and fermented foods, as well as healthy fats and lean protein sources, is vital to growing and maintaining a healthy, diverse range of gut bacteria.

When planning your intermittent diet, spare a thought for your influential gut bacteria and give them some goodness!

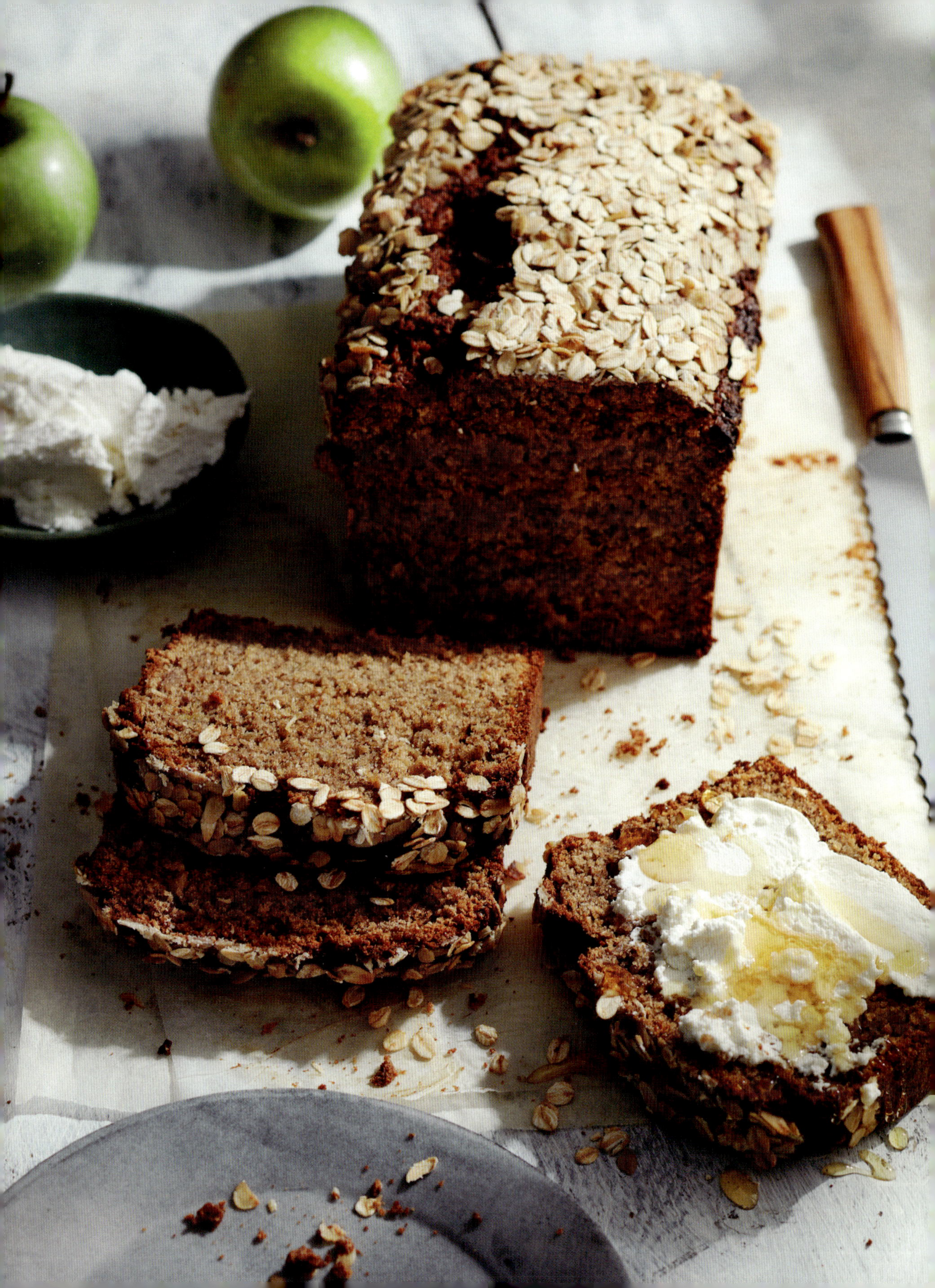

BIRCHER BANANA BREAD

PREP + COOK TIME *1 HOUR 40 MINUTES*
(+ OVERNIGHT REFRIGERATION & COOLING)
SERVES *12*

You will need to start this recipe a day ahead.

1 cup (170g) grated green apple

1 cup (280g) coconut yoghurt

1 cup (250ml) maple syrup, plus extra to serve

1 cup (280g) mashed over-ripe banana

1½ cups (135g) rolled oats

1 tbsp ground cinnamon

½ cup (125ml) extra virgin olive oil

½ cup (140g) tahini

2 extra-large eggs (60g each)

2⅓ cups (370g) wholemeal self-raising flour

1 tsp baking powder

½ cup (90g) firmly packed unrefined sugar (see tip)

labne or extra coconut yoghurt, to serve

1 To make bircher mixture, place apple, yoghurt, maple syrup, banana and 1 cup of the oats in a bowl; stir well to combine. Cover; refrigerate overnight.

2 Preheat oven to 160°C. Line base and sides of a 13cm x 25.5cm, 7.5cm deep loaf pan with two layers of baking paper, extending the papers 5cm over the edges.

3 Add cinnamon, oil, tahini and eggs to bircher mixture; stir to combine. Sift flour, baking powder and sugar onto bircher mixture, pushing sugar through the sieve using the back of a spoon; stir to combine well. Spoon mixture into loaf pan; smooth surface evenly. Sprinkle top with the remaining oats.

4 Bake bread for 1 hour. Cover loosely with foil to prevent overbrowning; bake for a further 25 minutes or until a skewer inserted into the centre comes out clean.

5 Cool bread in pan for 45 minutes. Using the paper as an aid, transfer bread from pan to a wire rack for 45 minutes or until cooled to room temperature.

6 Serve banana bread slices topped with labne and drizzled with extra maple syrup.

TIP Use any type of unrefined sugar such as rapadura or panela.

KEEPS Slice banana bread and wrap in individual portions. It will keep in an airtight container in the fridge for up to 1 week, or freezer for up to 1 month.

NUTRITION PER SERVING *25.3G TOTAL FAT (7.4G SATURATED FAT); 2253KJ (538 CAL); 65.3G CARBOHYDRATE; 10.3G PROTEIN; 7.4G FIBRE*

ROAST PUMPKIN DIP WITH SPICED CHICKPEAS

PREP + COOK TIME *1 HOUR*
SERVES *8 AS A STARTER*

1kg pumpkin, peeled, chopped coarsely

4 cloves garlic, unpeeled

2 tbsp extra virgin olive oil

2 tbsp tahini

½ cup (125ml) extra virgin olive oil, extra

2 tbsp red wine vinegar

MOUNTAIN BREAD CRISPS

200g wholemeal mountain bread

rice bran oil spray

1 tbsp sweet paprika

1 tbsp sesame seeds

SPICED CHICKPEAS

1 tbsp extra virgin olive oil

1 medium red onion (170g), halved, sliced

400g can chickpeas, drained, rinsed

1 clove garlic, sliced

2 tsp cumin seeds

1 tsp ground coriander

¼ tsp dried chilli flakes

1 tbsp pomegranate molasses

1 Preheat oven to 180°C. Line 2 large oven trays with baking paper.

2 Place pumpkin, garlic and oil on tray, then season; toss to coat well. Roast for 45 minutes or until tender; cool slightly.

3 Meanwhile, to make the mountain bread crisps, place half the bread between two oven trays; spray lightly with oil. Sprinkle with half the paprika and half the seeds; season lightly with salt and pepper. Bake for 10 minutes or until crisp. Repeat with remaining bread, paprika and seeds.

4 To make the spiced chickpeas, heat oil in a large frying pan over medium heat; cook onion, stirring occasionally, for 8 minutes or until soft. Add chickpeas and garlic; cook, stirring, for 3 minutes. Stir in spices and chilli; cook, stirring, for 1 minute or until fragrant. Stir in molasses; season to taste. Keep warm.

5 Squeeze garlic from skins into a large food processor. Add roasted pumpkin, tahini, extra oil and vinegar; process until smooth. Season to taste.

6 Spoon pumpkin mixture into a bowl; top with spiced chickpeas. Serve dip with mountain bread crisps.

DO-AHEAD Recipe can be prepared a day ahead; refrigerate dip and spiced chickpeas separately. Keep mountain bread crisps in an airtight container at room temperature. Reheat pumpkin mixture and spiced chickpeas just before serving.

NUTRITION PER SERVING *27.2G TOTAL FAT (4.1G SATURATED FAT); 1665KJ (398 CAL); 27G CARBOHYDRATE; 8.4G PROTEIN; 6.3G FIBRE*

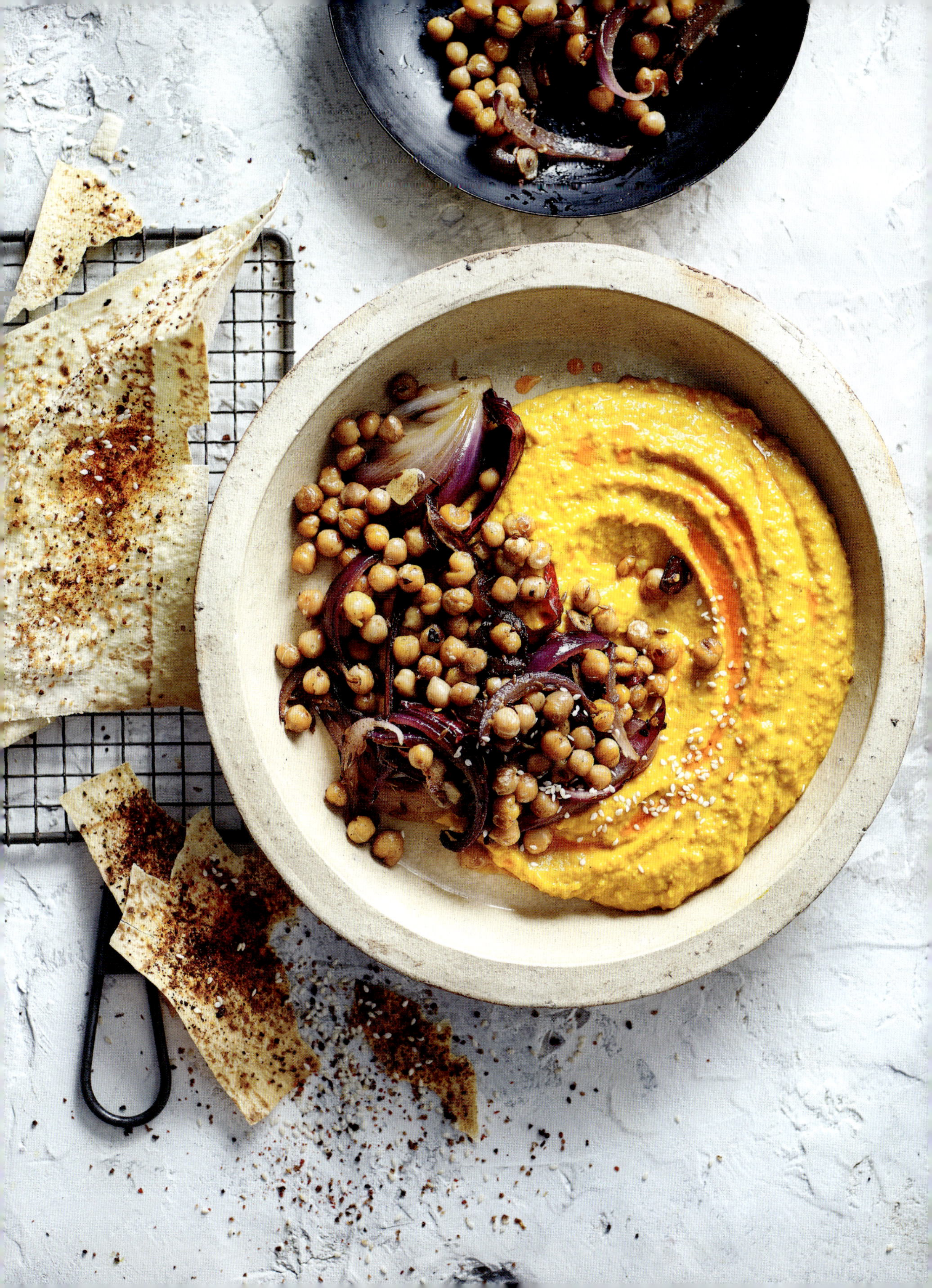

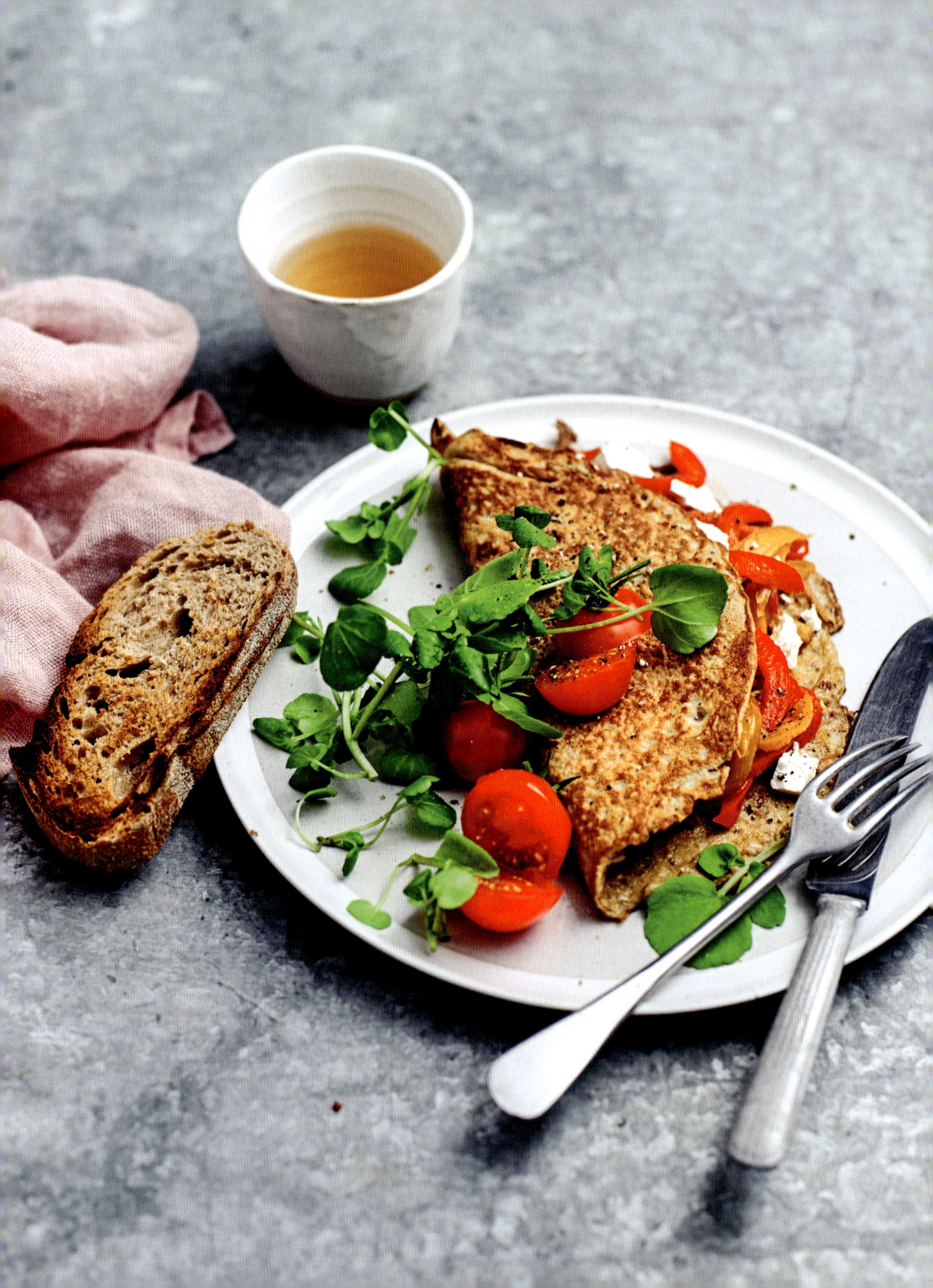

LENTIL OMELETTES WITH BRAISED CAPSICUM

PREP + COOK TIME *40 MINUTES*
SERVES *4*

1 tbsp extra virgin olive oil

1 medium red capsicum (200g), seeded, sliced thinly

2 medium yellow capsicums (400g), seeded, sliced thinly

1 long green chilli, sliced thinly

1½ tbsp red wine vinegar

6 extra-large eggs (60g each)

400g can lentils, drained, rinsed

1 tsp ground coriander

1 tsp ground cumin

⅓ cup (80ml) milk

2 tbsp soft fetta

200g cherry truss tomatoes, halved

60g trimmed watercress

4 slices wholemeal sourdough bread (45g each), toasted

1 Heat oil in a large heavy-based saucepan over low-medium heat. Cook capsicum, covered, stirring occasionally, for 15 minutes or until very soft and golden brown. Stir in chilli and vinegar; remove from heat.

2 Meanwhile, place eggs, lentils, spices and milk in a large bowl; season with pepper. Pulse with a stick blender (or use a small food processor) until almost smooth, with some coarsely crushed lentils still visible.

3 Heat a small frying pan over medium heat. Add a quarter of the egg mixture; cook for 2 minutes, using a spatula to pull egg inwards from edge of the pan towards the centre to create folds, letting raw egg mixture fill any gaps. Sprinkle a quarter of the capsicum mixture and 2 teaspoons fetta over one half of the omelette. Cook for 1 minute; flip uncovered half over top to cover capsicum mixture. Slide carefully onto a plate. Keep warm. Repeat three times with remaining egg mixture, capsicum mixture and fetta to make 4 omelettes in total.

4 Top omelettes with tomatoes and watercress; season. Serve with toast.

NUTRITION PER SERVING *15.6G TOTAL FAT (4.7G SATURATED FAT); 1376KJ (328 CAL); 21.9G CARBOHYDRATE; 21.5G PROTEIN; 6.5G FIBRE*

BLACK BEAN CHILLI WITH GUACAMOLE & CORN CHIPS

PREP + COOK TIME *40 MINUTES*
SERVES *4*

olive oil spray

1 large red onion (300g), diced finely

1 medium red capsicum (200g), seeded, diced finely

1 large carrot (180g), chopped finely

3 celery stalks (450g), trimmed, chopped finely

2 cloves garlic, crushed

2 tsp ground cumin

2 tsp Mexican seasoning

1 tbsp tomato paste

400g can diced tomatoes

400g can black beans, drained, rinsed

3 slices corn mountain bread (75g), cut into 12 triangles each (see tip)

⅓ cup (40g) grated reduced-fat tasty cheese

½ cup (140g) plain yoghurt

½ cup coriander leaves

1 lime (65g), cut into wedges

GUACAMOLE

1 small avocado (200g)

¼ cup (70g) plain yoghurt

3 tsp lime juice

1 Spray a large heavy-based saucepan with oil; heat over medium heat. Add onion, capsicum, carrot and celery; cook, stirring, for 5 minutes or until onion softens.

2 Add garlic and spices to pan; cook, stirring, for 1 minute. Add tomato paste; cook, stirring, for a further 1 minute. Add tomatoes, black beans and 1 cup (250ml) water; bring to the boil. Reduce heat to low; cook, covered, stirring occasionally, for 20 minutes or until vegetables soften.

3 Meanwhile, preheat oven to 200°C.

4 To make guacamole, mash ingredients in a small bowl until smooth.

5 Place mountain bread triangles on an oven tray. Place in oven for 5 minutes or until light golden and crisp.

6 Evenly divide black bean chilli, guacamole, corn chips, cheese and yoghurt among four bowls; sprinkle with coriander and season with pepper. Serve with lime wedges.

TIP Making your own corn chips from corn mountain bread makes this a healthier option than using regular corn chips. Each mountain bread slice will yield 12 triangles (36 in total), which is 9 chips per serve.

NUTRITION PER SERVING *15G TOTAL FAT (5G SATURATED FAT); 1571KJ (375 CAL); 33.3G CARBOHYDRATE; 17.7G PROTEIN; 14.6G FIBRE*

PREP IT
Portion chilli and guacamole separately; refrigerate for up to 4 days.

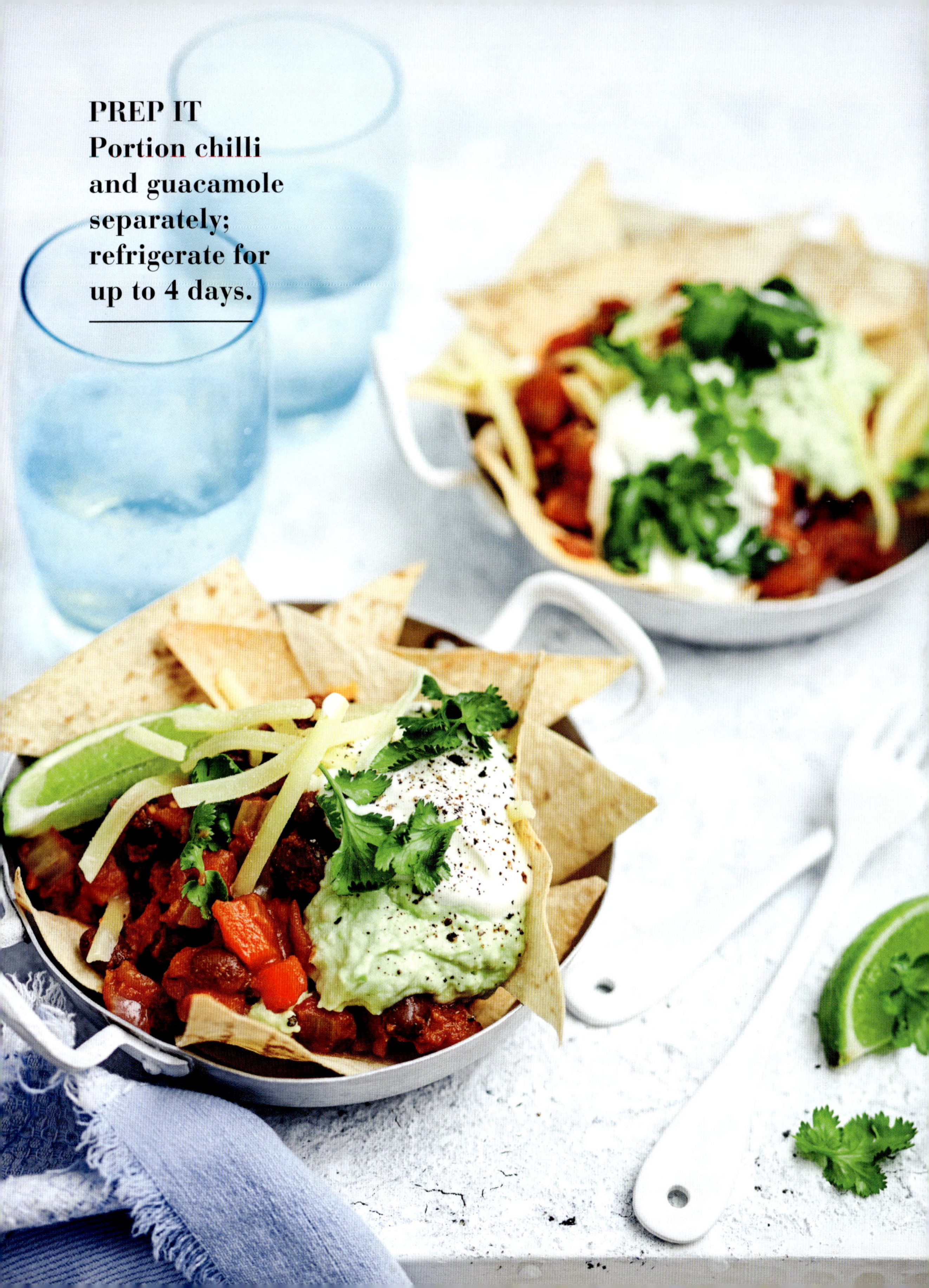

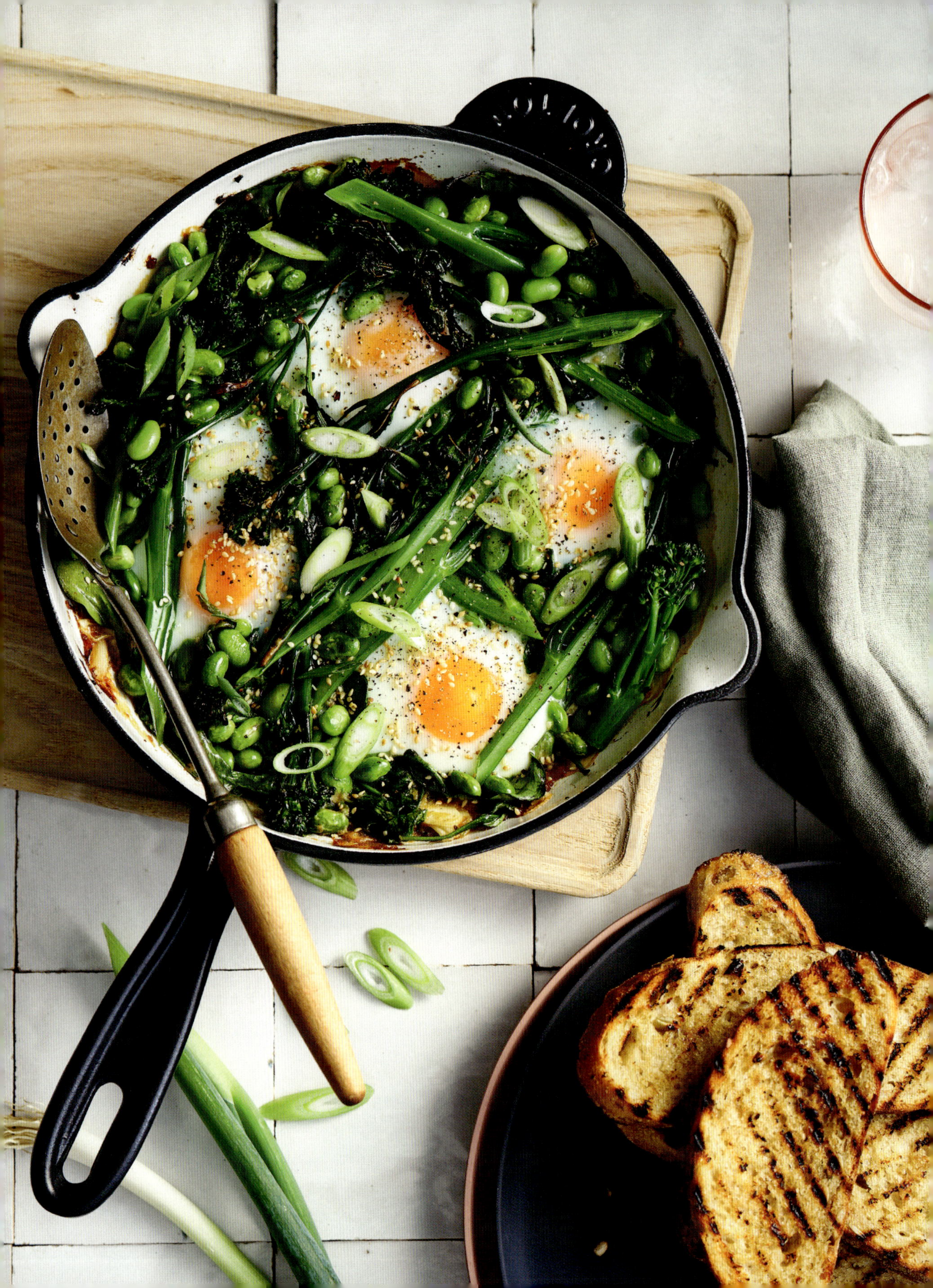

BAKED EGGS WITH GREENS & MISO

PREP + COOK TIME *25 MINUTES*
SERVES *4*

- **1 bunch broccolini (175g), trimmed, halved lengthways**
- **1 cup (150g) frozen shelled edamame**
- **1 tbsp sesame oil**
- **2 tsp finely grated fresh ginger**
- **2 cloves garlic, sliced thinly**
- **3 green onions, sliced thinly**
- **¼ cup (60g) white (shiro) miso paste**
- **1 tbsp mirin**
- **120g baby spinach leaves**
- **4 extra-large eggs (60g each)**
- **1 tsp sesame seeds**
- **4 slices rye bread (260g)**

1 Preheat oven to 200°C.

2 Cook broccolini and edamame in a medium saucepan of salted boiling water for 2 minutes or until tender-crisp. Drain; refresh under cold running water.

3 Heat 2 teaspoons of the sesame oil in a large ovenproof frying pan. Cook ginger, garlic and two-thirds of the green onion, stirring, for 2 minutes or until soft.

4 Add miso and mirin to pan; stir to combine. Add spinach and 1 tablespoon water; cook spinach for 30 seconds or until wilted.

5 Stir in broccolini and edamame. Using the back of a spoon, make four equally spaced indents in vegetable mixture. Crack eggs into hollows, then sprinkle with sesame seeds. Season well.

6 Transfer pan to oven; bake vegetables and eggs for 10 minutes or until eggs are just set.

7 Meanwhile, brush bread slices with remaining sesame oil. Chargrill bread, in batches, for 1 minute each side or until grill marks appear.

8 Top vegetables and eggs with remaining green onion and serve with charred bread.

TIP Instead of chargrilling the bread, you can toast in a toaster and then brush with sesame oil.

SWAP You can use peas instead of the edamame, if preferred.

NUTRITION PER SERVING *13.2G TOTAL FAT (2.45G SATURATED FAT); 1508KJ (361 CAL); 36.5G CARBOHYDRATE; 19.2G PROTEIN; 9.3G FIBRE*

SPANAKOPITA QUESADILLAS

PREP + COOK TIME *35 MINUTES*
SERVES *4*

- **2 tsp extra virgin olive oil**
- **1 small red onion (100g), chopped finely**
- **1 clove garlic, crushed**
- **200g baby spinach leaves, chopped coarsely**
- **2 extra-large eggs (60g each), beaten lightly**
- **100g reduced-fat fetta, crumbled**
- **1½ tbsp finely grated parmesan**
- **2 tsp finely grated lemon rind**
- **⅓ cup chopped dill**
- **4 wholegrain tortillas (160g)**
- **1 Lebanese cucumber (130g), chopped**
- **250g cherry tomatoes, halved**
- **⅓ cup (95g) store-bought tzatziki**
- **1 medium lemon (140g), cut into wedges**

1 Heat oil in a large heavy-based non-stick frying pan over medium heat. Cook onion, garlic and spinach, stirring, for 2 minutes or until softened. Transfer to a large bowl; allow to cool slightly. Wipe pan clean with paper towel.

2 Add egg, fetta, parmesan, lemon rind and 2 tablespoons of the dill to spinach mixture. Season; whisk to combine.

3 Heat frying pan over low heat. Spread a quarter of the spinach mixture over one half of a tortilla; fold over to enclose. Repeat with remaining spinach mixture and tortillas. Cook quesadillas, in batches, for 3 minutes each side or until warmed through and golden.

4 Combine cucumber, tomatoes and remaining dill in a medium bowl; season with pepper.

5 Cut quesadillas into triangles. Serve with cucumber salad, tzatziki and lemon wedges.

PREP IT Quesadillas can be made a day ahead up to the end of step 3; store, covered, the fridge. Reheat in a large frying pan, over low heat.

NUTRITION PER PORTION *13.4G TOTAL FAT (5.2G SATURATED FAT); 1236KJ (295 CAL); 24.3G CARBOHYDRATE; 16.6G PROTEIN; 4.8G FIBRE*

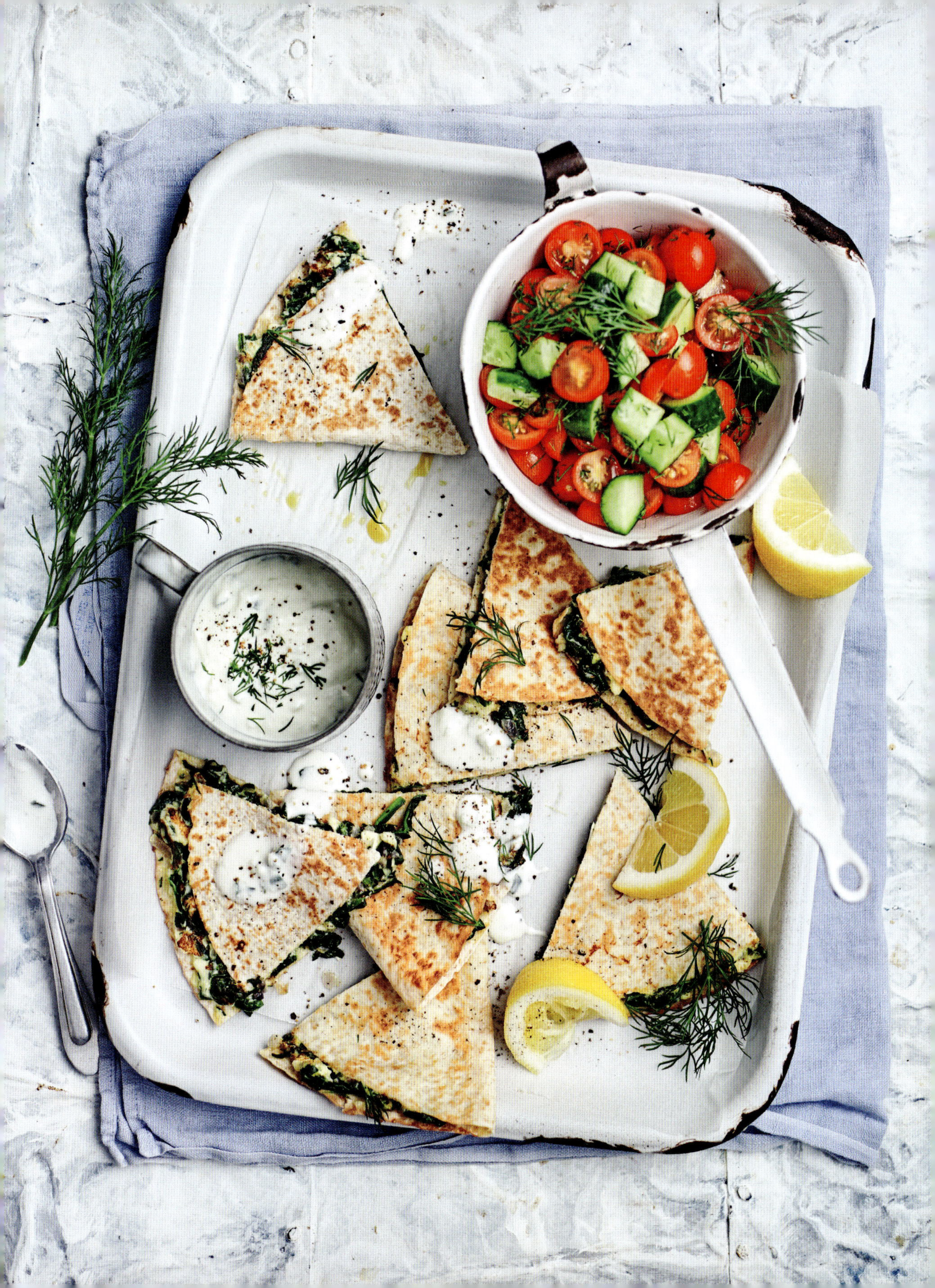

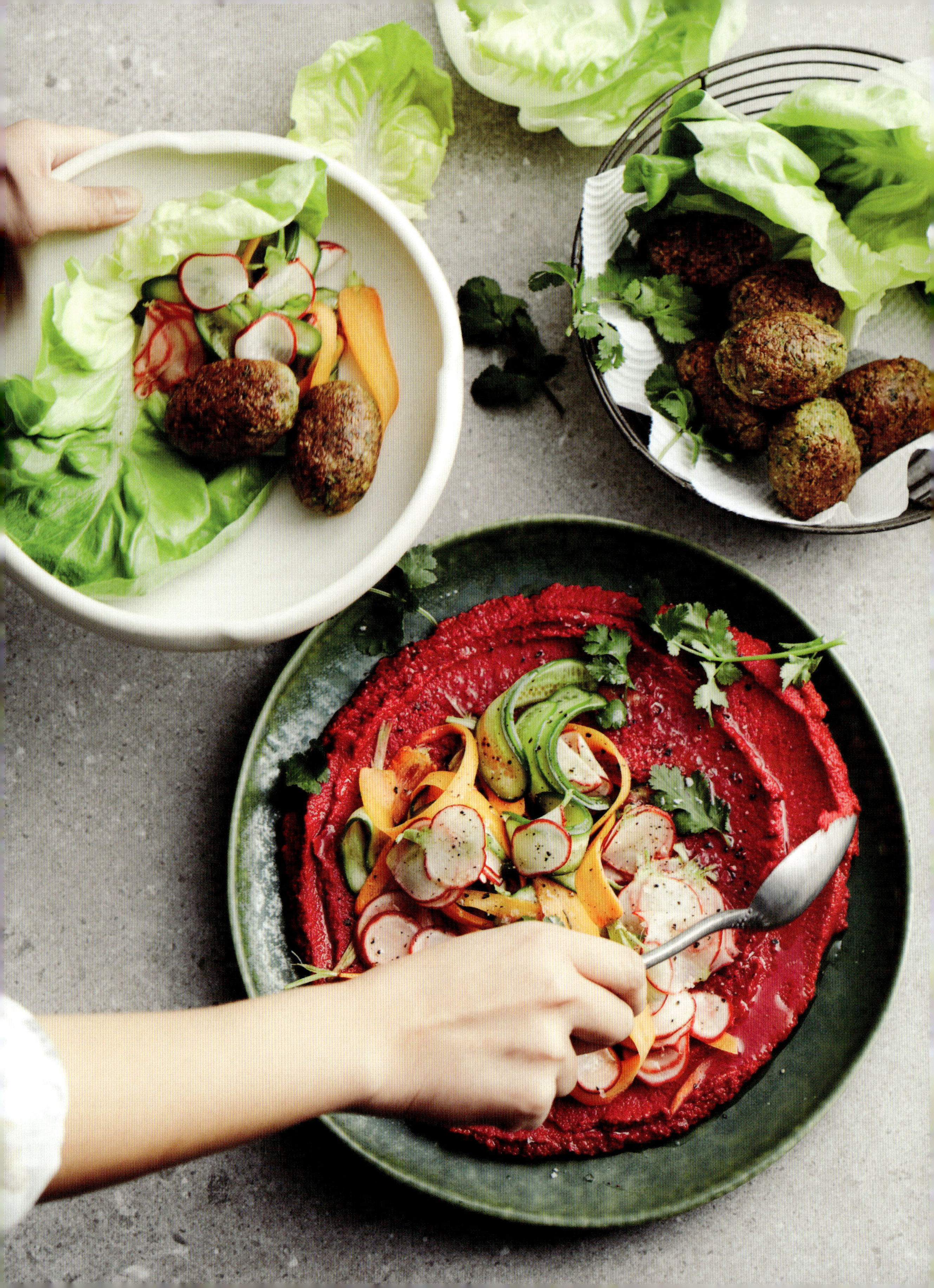

QUINOA FALAFEL WITH PICKLED VEG & BEETROOT HUMMUS

PREP + COOK TIME *35 MINUTES*
SERVES 4

400g can chickpeas, drained, rinsed

½ cup (40g) quinoa flakes

2 tsp ground cumin

2 tsp ground coriander

4 green onions, chopped

1 long green chilli, chopped

½ cup finely chopped coriander leaves and stems

1 tbsp golden linseed meal (flaxmeal)

¼ cup (60ml) extra virgin olive oil

4 leaves butter lettuce

PICKLED VEGETABLES

5 baby cucumbers (150g)

5 red radishes (175g)

4 baby carrots (80g)

½ cup (125ml) white wine vinegar

2 tbsp honey

BEETROOT HUMMUS

1 medium beetroot (175g), grated coarsely

400g can chickpeas, drained, rinsed

1 clove garlic, crushed

¼ cup (60ml) lemon juice

1 tsp ground cumin

1 To make pickled vegetables, thinly slice cucumber, radishes and carrot lengthways, using using a mandoline or very sharp knife. Combine vegetables with vinegar and honey in a glass or stainless steel bowl. Refrigerate for 30 minutes. Drain.

2 Meanwhile, to make beetroot hummus, process ingredients until smooth. Season. (Makes 2 cups.)

3 Process chickpeas, quinoa flakes, spices, green onion, chilli, coriander and linseed meal in cleaned food processor until combined. Divide mixture into 8 portions; shape each into a 4cm x 6cm oval falafel.

4 Heat oil in a large non-stick frying pan over medium heat; cook falafels for 4 minutes, turning, until golden.

5 Spread beetroot hummus over the base of a shallow bowl and top with pickled vegetables. Serve with lettuce leaves and falafel.

NUTRITION PER SERVING *18.9G TOTAL FAT (2.6G SATURATED FAT); 1761KJ (421 CAL); 43.1G CARBOHYDRATE; 12.3G PROTEIN; 13.6G FIBRE*

ASIAN GREENS & TOFU WITH GREEN TEA NOODLE SALAD

PREP + COOK TIME *25 MINUTES*
SERVES *4*

4 extra-large eggs (60g each)

150g green tea soba noodles

1 tbsp sesame oil

2 tbsp finely grated fresh ginger

2 tsp tamari

1 tbsp rice wine vinegar

2 tbsp wakame (dried seaweed) (see tip)

1 tsp white (shiro) miso paste

400g firm tofu, cut into 1cm thick slices

2 bunches gai lan (1kg), trimmed

2 green onions, sliced thinly

½ cup coriander leaves

½ long red chilli, sliced thinly

2 tsp black sesame seeds

1 Bring eggs to the boil in a small saucepan of water over high heat. Boil for 4 minutes. Cool under cold running water. Peel, halve and reserve.

2 Meanwhile, cook noodles according to packet directions. Reserve 1 tablespoon of cooking water. Drain, rinse; drain well.

3 Combine 2 teaspoons of the sesame oil and 1 tablespoon of the ginger, the tamari, vinegar and 1 tablespoon water in a small jug. Season with pepper.

4 Combine noodles, half the ginger dressing, the wakame and reserved cooking water in a bowl.

5 Spread miso and remaining ginger over tofu. Heat remaining sesame oil in a large frying pan over medium-low heat; cook tofu for 4 minutes each side until golden. Transfer to a plate. Heat same pan to high heat; add gai lan and 2 tablespoons water; cook, stirring, for 3 minutes or until just tender. Add remaining ginger dressing to gai lan; remove from heat.

6 Divide noodle mixture among serving bowls; top with gai lan, tofu, green onion, coriander, chilli, halved egg and black sesame seeds.

TIP Dried seaweed (wakame) is available from Asian food stores. It has a much lower sodium content than dried nori sheets.

NUTRITION PER SERVING *20.1G TOTAL FAT (3G SATURATED FAT); 1922KJ (459 CAL); 46.7G CARBOHYDRATE; 26.5G PROTEIN; 13.3G FIBRE*

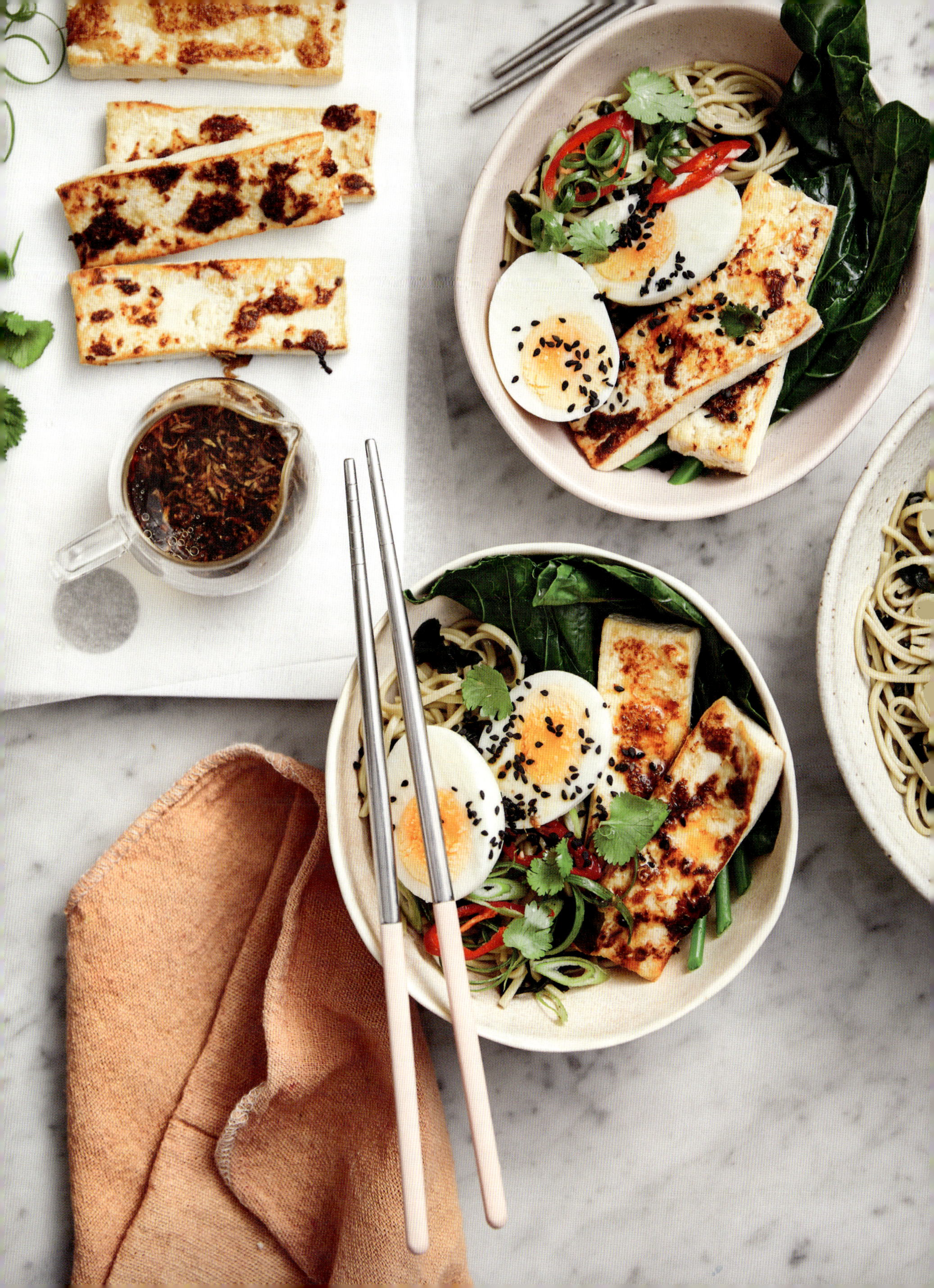

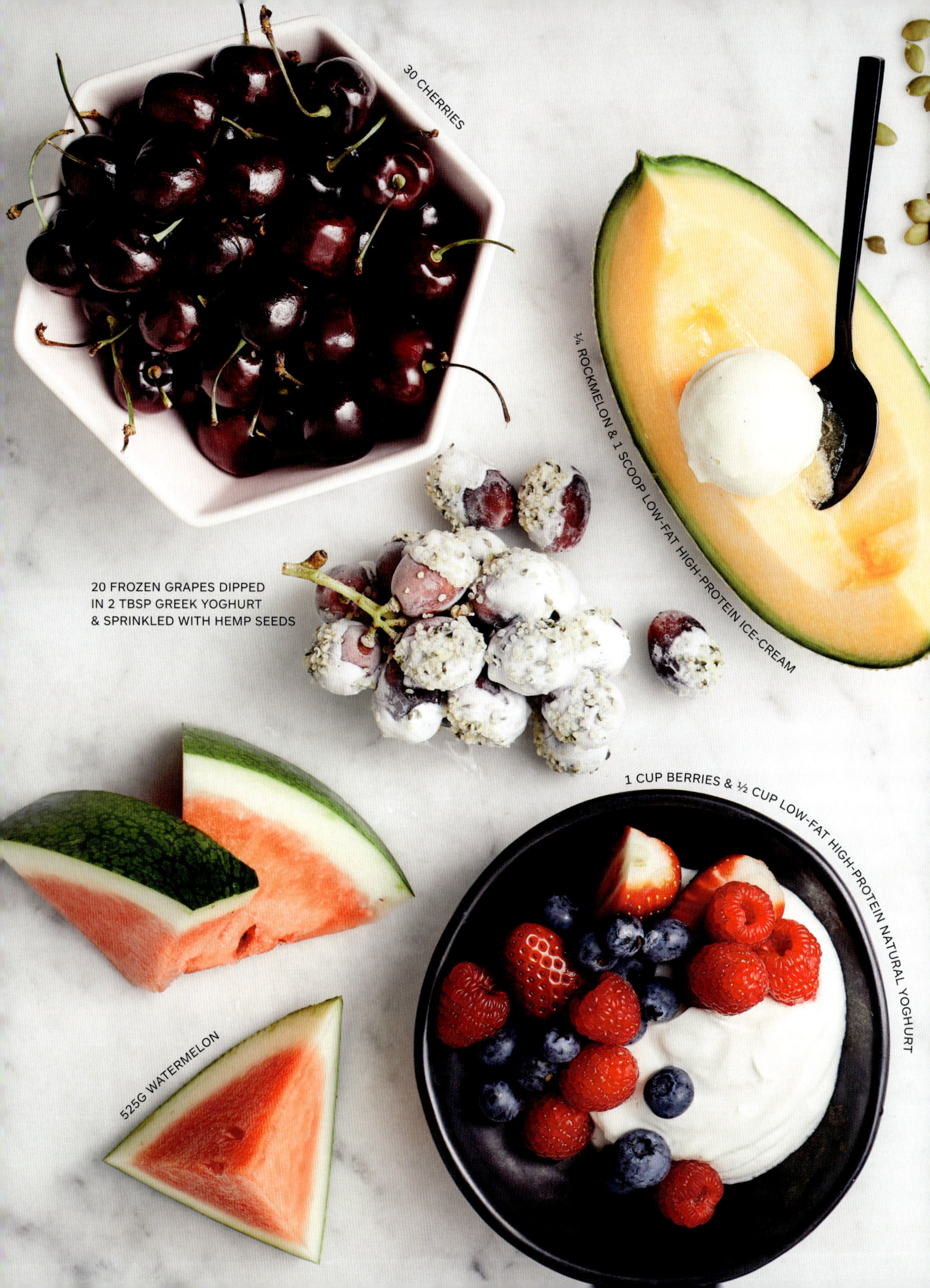
30 CHERRIES
¼ ROCKMELON & 1 SCOOP LOW-FAT HIGH-PROTEIN ICE-CREAM
20 FROZEN GRAPES DIPPED
IN 2 TBSP GREEK YOGHURT
& SPRINKLED WITH HEMP SEEDS
1 CUP BERRIES & ½ CUP LOW-FAT HIGH-PROTEIN NATURAL YOGHURT
525G WATERMELON

SNACK IDEAS

SWEET

¼ CUP PEPITAS &
NATURAL ALMONDS
1 PEACH
CHOCOLATE PUDDING: ½ CUP COTTAGE CHEESE, 1 TSP COCOA POWDER
& 1 TSP MAPLE SYRUP
25G DARK 70% CHOCOLATE
1 BANANA
2 RYVITA MULTIGRAIN CRACKERS,
3 TSP LITE CREAM CHEESE &
1 SLICED KIWIFRUIT

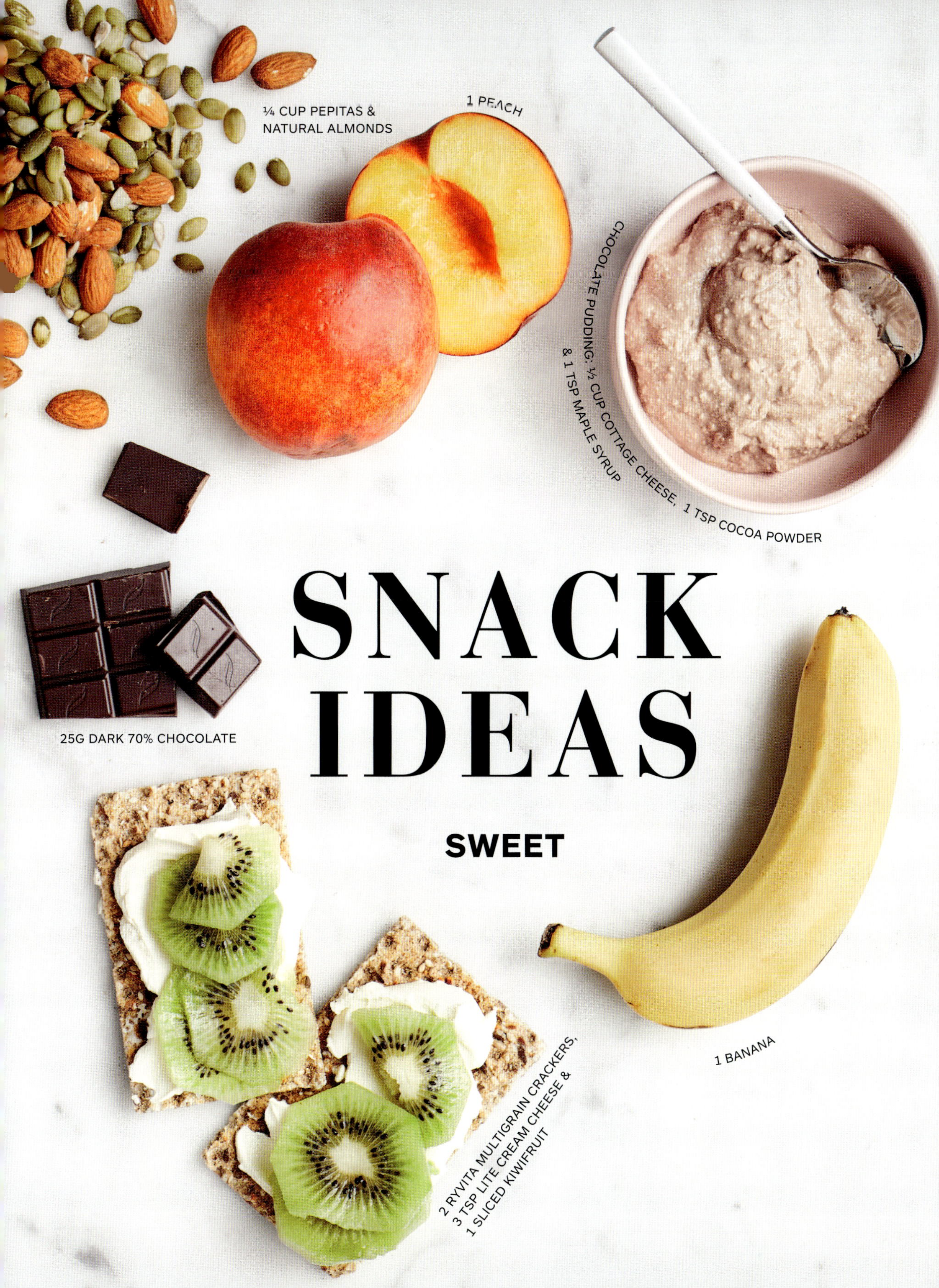

GREEN MINESTRONE

PREP + COOK TIME *35 MINUTES*
SERVES *4*

2 tbsp extra virgin olive oil

1 tsp finely chopped sage

2 cloves garlic, chopped finely

1 medium leek (350g), chopped finely

1 medium parsnip (250g), cut into 1cm cubes

2 trimmed celery stalks (200g), sliced thinly

150g kale, stems discarded, torn in pieces

1.5 litres (6 cups) vegetable stock

150g green beans, trimmed, cut into 1cm lengths

2 medium zucchini (240g), halved, sliced thinly

400g can cannellini beans, drained, rinsed

PESTO

2 cups basil leaves

⅓ cup (25g) grated parmesan

¼ cup (40g) pine nuts, toasted

½ clove garlic, peeled

½ cup (125ml) extra virgin olive oil

1 Heat oil in a large saucepan over medium heat. Cook sage, garlic and leek, stirring, for 3 minutes or until leek is soft. Add parsnip, celery and kale to pan; cook, stirring, for a further 2 minutes or until kale is bright green. Add stock; bring to the boil. Reduce heat to low; simmer, for 15 minutes or until the parsnip is almost tender.

2 Add green beans, zucchini and cannellini beans; simmer for a further 5 minutes or until zucchini is just tender. Season to taste.

3 Meanwhile, to make pesto, blend or process ingredients until smooth. Transfer to a small bowl; season to taste.

4 Serve soup topped with pesto.

TIP Cut the leek in half lengthways and rinse carefully between the layers; they can be quite gritty.

DO-AHEAD Soup can be made a day ahead; keep covered in the fridge. Pesto can be made 3 days ahead; keep tightly covered, in a airtight container, in the fridge. Soup and pesto can be frozen separately, for up to 3 months.

NUTRITION PER SERVING *48.8G TOTAL FAT (8G SATURATED FAT); 2614KJ (625 CAL); 23.6G CARBOHYDRATE; 15G PROTEIN; 15G FIBRE*

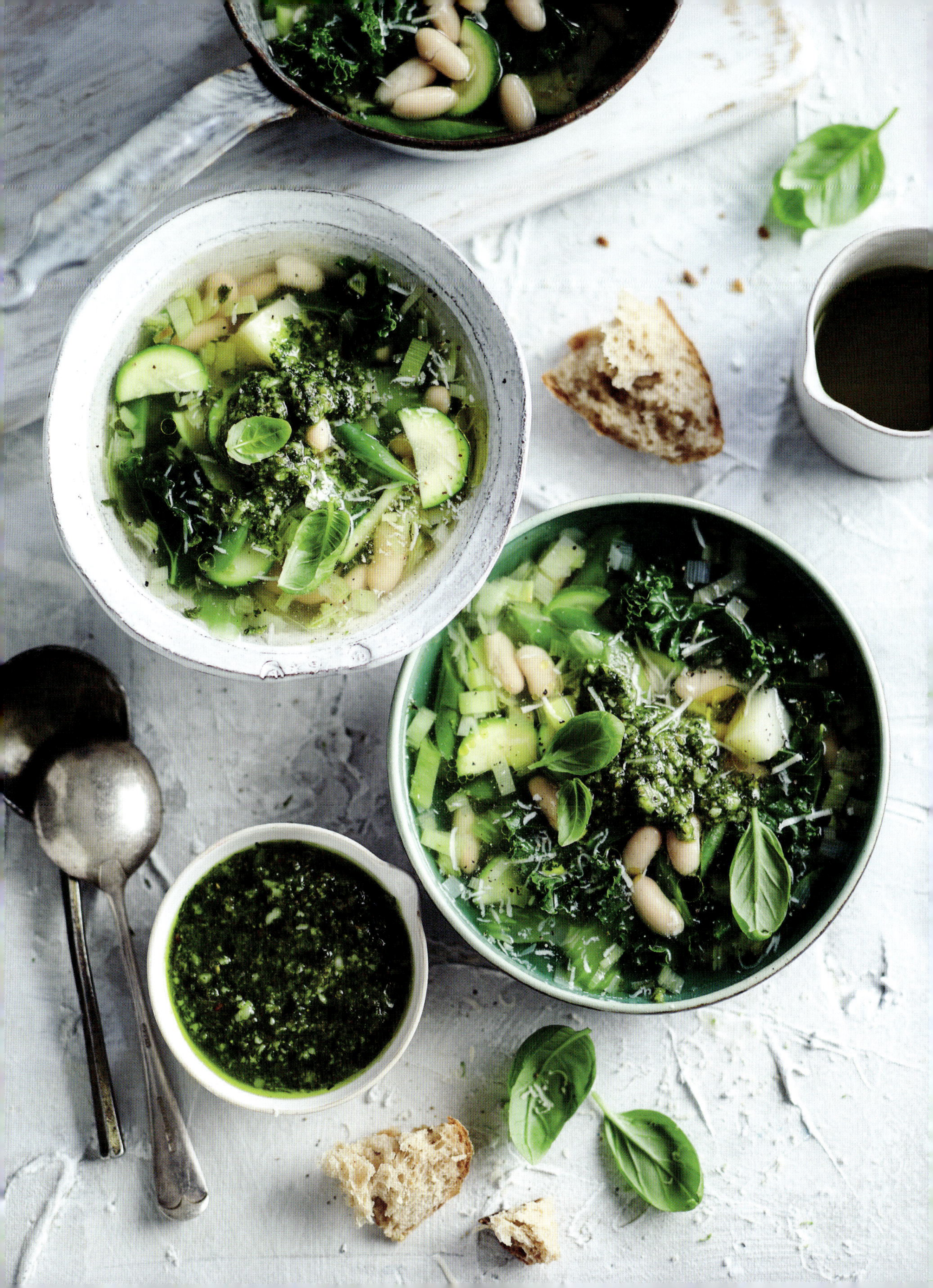

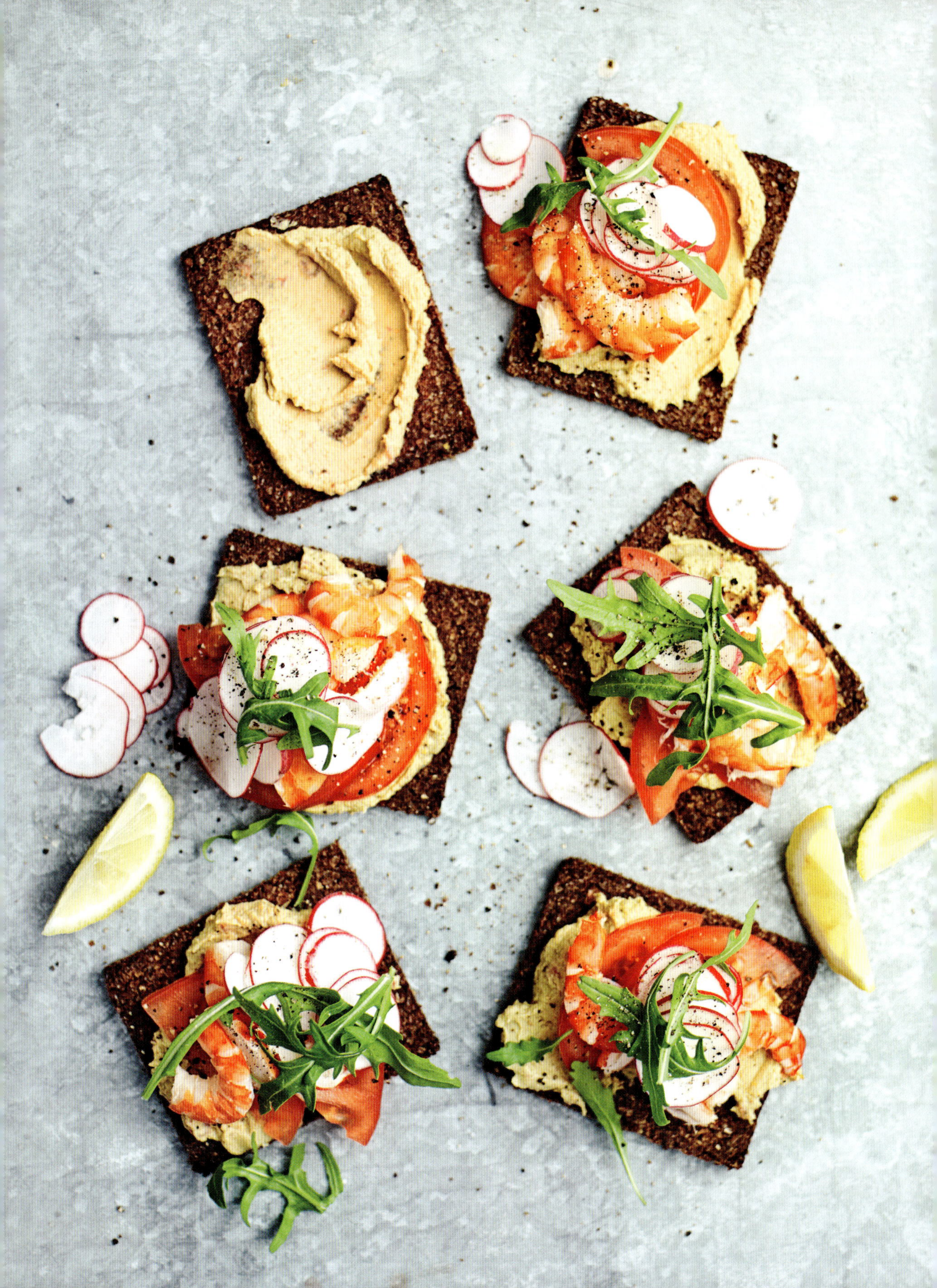

PUMPERNICKEL WITH SMOKY TOMATO LIPTAUER

PREP + COOK TIME *30 MINUTES*
SERVES *4*

- **300g pumpernickel bread**
- **¾ cup (180g) reduced-fat soft ricotta**
- **2 tbsp semi-dried tomatoes (see tips), chopped coarsely**
- **1 tbsp chopped chives**
- **2 tsp lemon juice**
- **¼ tsp smoked paprika**
- **1 large tomato (220g), halved, sliced thinly**
- **400g medium prawns, peeled, deveined, halved lengthways**
- **6 small radishes (90g), sliced thinly**
- **40g baby rocket leaves**
- **1 medium lemon (140g), cut into wedges**

1 Preheat oven to 200°C. Line an oven tray with baking paper.

2 Place pumpernickel on the tray; bake, turning halfway through baking time, for 20 minutes or until crisp.

3 Meanwhile, to make liptauer, blend or process ricotta, semi-dried tomato, chives, lemon juice and paprika until well combined. Season to taste.

4 Spread liptauer on pumpernickel slices. Top with tomato, prawns, radishes and rocket. Serve with lemon wedges.

TIPS We used the semi-dried tomatoes not packed in oil. To save time, simply spread the liptauer on untoasted pumpernickel bread.

PREP IT You can make the liptauer a day ahead. Cover and refrigerate until ready to serve.

NUTRITION PER SERVING *3.7G TOTAL FAT (1.3G SATURATED FAT); 1213KJ (289 CAL); 36.4G CARBOHYDRATE; 21.9G PROTEIN; 7.7G FIBRE*

BLACK-EYED BEAN & MUSHROOM BURGERS

PREP + COOK TIME *30 MINUTES (+ COOLING & REFRIGERATION)*
SERVES 4

⅓ cup (80ml) extra virgin olive oil

1 small onion (80g), chopped finely

300g mushrooms, quartered (see tips)

2 tbsp thyme leaves

400g can black-eyed beans, drained, rinsed

1 extra-large egg (60g), beaten lightly

1 cup (80g) finely grated parmesan

2 cloves garlic, crushed

⅔ cup (70g) mixed grain packaged breadcrumbs

100g cabbage, sliced thinly

2 tbsp lemon juice

4 x 85g white milk baps

⅓ cup (100g) whole-egg mayonnaise

1 small bulb fennel (200g), shaved thinly, fronds reserved

1 tbsp hot chilli sauce

1 Heat 2 tablespoons of the oil in a frying pan over medium heat; cook onion, mushrooms and thyme, stirring, for 10 minutes or until softened and lightly golden. Cool.

2 Place mushroom mixture and beans in a food processor; pulse until chopped coarsely. Transfer mixture to a medium bowl; stir in egg, parmesan, garlic and breadcrumbs. Season. Shape mixture into four patties; place on a plate. Cover; refrigerate for 30 minutes.

3 Heat remaining oil in same frying pan over medium heat; cook patties for 3 minutes each side, turning carefully, or until browned and heated through.

4 Meanwhile, combine cabbage and lemon juice in a large bowl; season to taste.

5 Cut milk baps in half horizontally. Spread bap bases with mayonnaise; top with fennel, fennel fronds, patties, chilli sauce, cabbage mixture and bap tops.

TIPS We used half button mushrooms and half Swiss brown mushrooms. For a stronger mushroom flavour, use cup or flat mushrooms instead of buttons. If the fennel doesn't have fronds, use dill, or just omit it.

DO-AHEAD Patties can be made a day ahead; keep covered in the fridge.

NUTRITION PER SERVING *45.4G TOTAL FAT (9.9G SATURATED FAT); 3432KJ (820 CAL); 69.1G CARBOHYDRATE; 27.2G PROTEIN; 11.9G FIBRE*

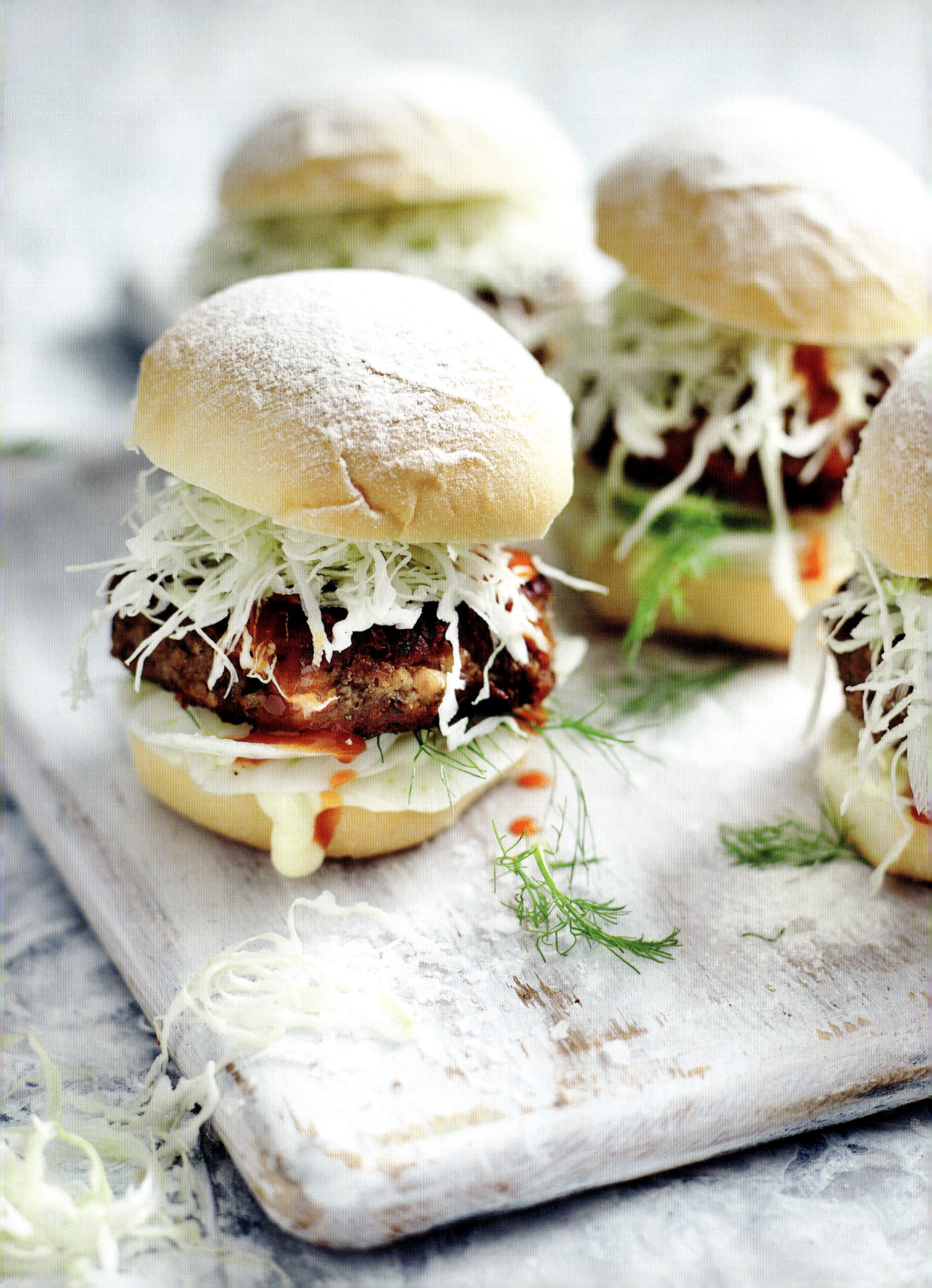

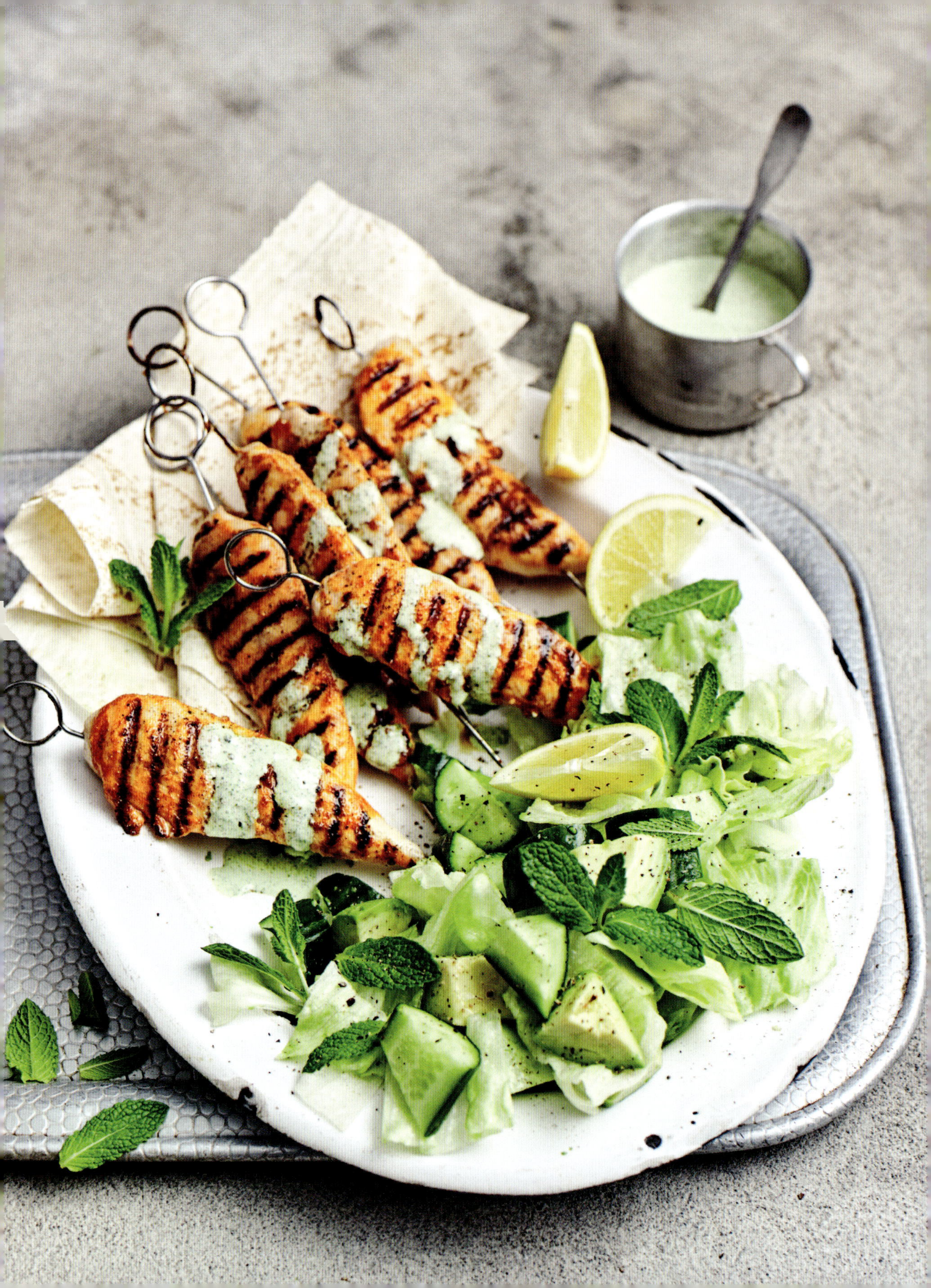

SPICY CHICKEN, LETTUCE & AVOCADO WRAPS

PREP + COOK TIME *20 MINUTES*
SERVES 4

- **500g chicken tenderloins**
- **¼ cup (60ml) sambal chilli sauce (see tips)**
- **⅔ cup (190g) Greek yoghurt**
- **2 cups mint leaves**
- **½ large iceberg lettuce (350g), chopped coarsely**
- **2 Lebanese cucumbers (260g), chopped coarsely**
- **1 small avocado (200g), chopped coarsely**
- **2 tbsp lemon juice**
- **4 slices mountain bread (100g)**
- **1 medium lemon (140g), cut into wedges**

1 Place chicken and chilli sauce in a medium bowl; mix to coat chicken well. Thread chicken onto skewers; place on a tray lined with plastic wrap.

2 To make yoghurt sauce, process yoghurt and 1 cup of the mint until smooth. Transfer to a small bowl, cover; refrigerate until ready to serve.

3 Heat a grill plate (or grill pan) over medium heat; line with baking paper. Cook chicken skewers for 3 minutes each side or until charred and cooked through. Transfer to a plate; cover loosely with foil to keep warm.

4 Meanwhile, place lettuce, cucumber, avocado, remaining mint and lemon juice in a large bowl. Toss gently to combine.

5 Divide chicken, salad and yoghurt sauce among bread wraps; serve with lemon wedges.

TIPS You need 8 skewers for this recipe. You can use either metal or bamboo skewers. We used sambal asli, a Malaysian-style chilli sauce, but your favourite chilli sauce would work just as well.

DO-AHEAD The chicken can be marinated 1 day ahead; store, covered, in the fridge.

NUTRITION PER SERVING *11.9G TOTAL FAT (3.4G SATURATED FAT); 1552KJ (370 CAL); 27.3G CARBOHYDRATE; 34.6G PROTEIN; 5.4G FIBRE*

HAM & GREEN ONION FRITTERS

PREP + COOK TIME *20 MINUTES*
SERVES *4*

250g red grape tomatoes

1 tsp balsamic vinegar

1½ tbsp extra virgin olive oil

1 cup (135g) gluten-free self-raising flour

¾ cup (180ml) soy milk

250g gluten-free shaved ham, chopped finely

4 green onions, sliced thinly

1 large avocado (320g), chopped

lemon wedges, to serve

1 Preheat oven to 200°C.

2 Place tomatoes on an oven tray; drizzle with vinegar and 1 teaspoon of the oil. Season. Roast for 15 minutes or until tomatoes just soften.

3 Sift flour into a large bowl. Gradually add milk, in batches, stirring after each addition. Add ham and green onion; stir to combine. Season.

4 Heat remaining oil in a frying pan over medium heat. Spoon ¼-cups of batter into pan; cook for 2½ minutes each side or until golden brown and cooked through. Repeat with remaining batter to make 8 fritters in total.

5 Top warm fritters with avocado and roasted tomatoes; serve with lemon wedges.

TIP Make these gluten- and dairy-free fritters meat free by swapping the ham for edamame (soy beans).

PREP IT Divide cooked tomatoes and fritters into 4 portions. Refrigerate for up to 4 days. Reheat and serve with avocado.

NUTRITION PER SERVING *24.8G TOTAL FAT (5.6G SATURATED FAT); 1822KJ (435 CAL); 31.5G CARBOHYDRATE; 20.1G PROTEIN; 4G FIBRE*

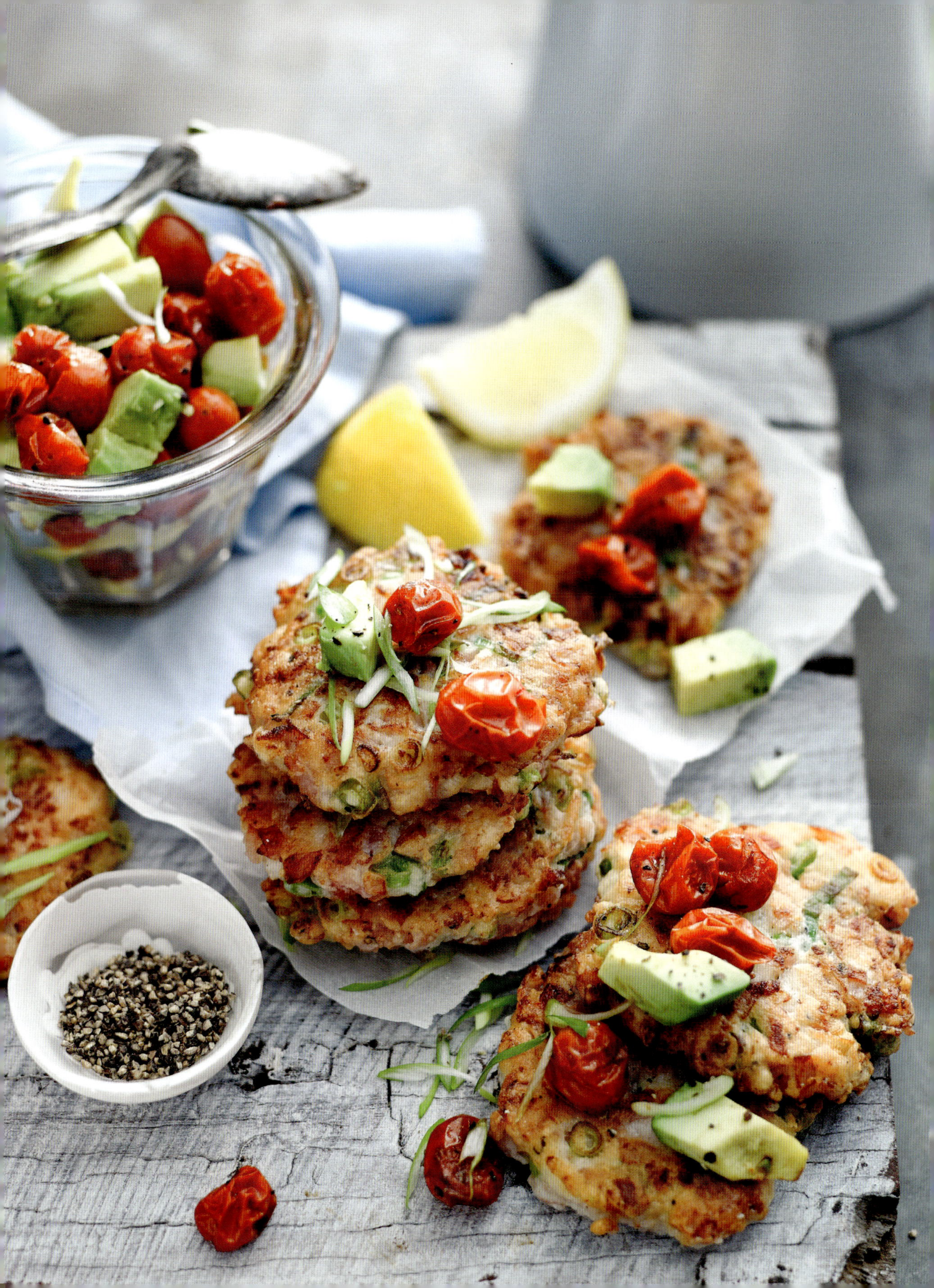

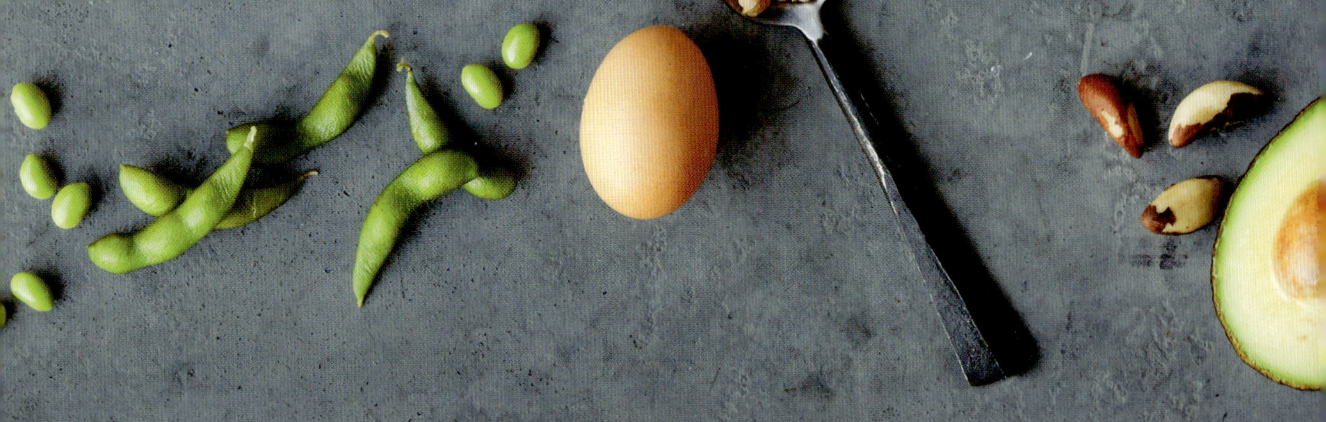

MEAL PREP

While we all have good intentions to eat healthily, road blocks such as lack of time and energy, and work, frequently conspire to make us crumple at the first hurdle and order takeaway.

This is where the practice of meal prepping can assist and set you on a path to better eating habits, especially when time challenged. Homemade meals are much easier to achieve if there is a degree of planning behind them, from knowing what you are going to eat, to starting the prep for it, or completing the entire meal ahead of time.

Restaurant chefs have always employed a practice called 'mise en place', a French culinary term which simply means 'everything in its place'. It's a practical system of preparing foods in advance, depending on the ingredient and recipe, it can be a simple as having ingredients peeled and chopped, having the base recipes cooked or even completed meals ready for reheating. This allows chefs to prepare meals quickly, even where they may not know in advance how many mouths they have to feed.

Planning your shopping and meal prepping will help you from entering a food rut and critically derailing your healthy eating plan.

Ensure the kitchen is always well stocked; dedicate time each week to preparing a weekly menu and shopping list. This way you are not pressed to think of what to cook after a busy tiring day. Sunday is often a good day for full-time workers to jump into the kitchen and make a head start on the upcoming week's cooking. If Sundays are taken, instead aim to meal prep on Monday or mid-week.

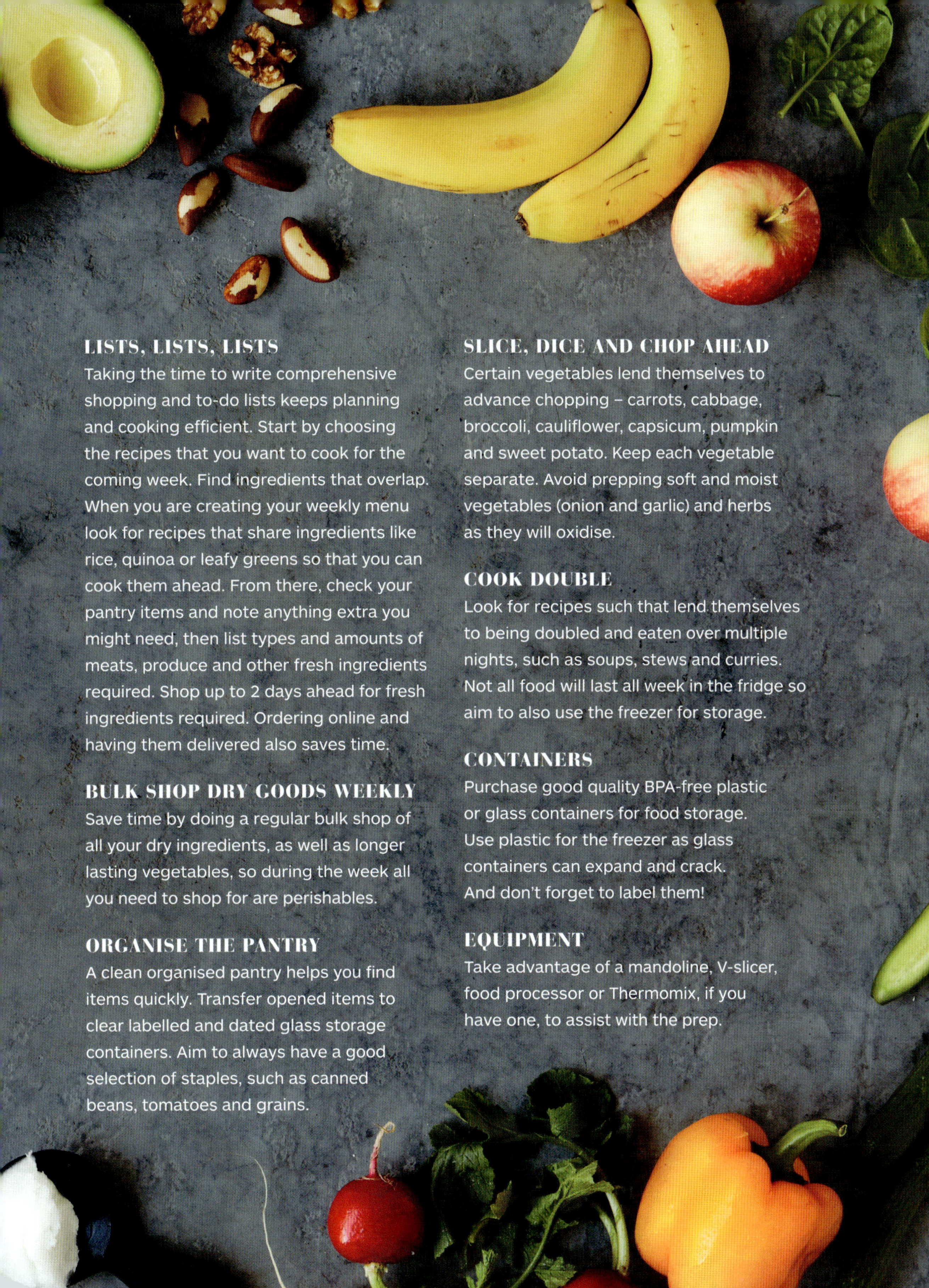

LISTS, LISTS, LISTS

Taking the time to write comprehensive shopping and to-do lists keeps planning and cooking efficient. Start by choosing the recipes that you want to cook for the coming week. Find ingredients that overlap. When you are creating your weekly menu look for recipes that share ingredients like rice, quinoa or leafy greens so that you can cook them ahead. From there, check your pantry items and note anything extra you might need, then list types and amounts of meats, produce and other fresh ingredients required. Shop up to 2 days ahead for fresh ingredients required. Ordering online and having them delivered also saves time.

BULK SHOP DRY GOODS WEEKLY

Save time by doing a regular bulk shop of all your dry ingredients, as well as longer lasting vegetables, so during the week all you need to shop for are perishables.

ORGANISE THE PANTRY

A clean organised pantry helps you find items quickly. Transfer opened items to clear labelled and dated glass storage containers. Aim to always have a good selection of staples, such as canned beans, tomatoes and grains.

SLICE, DICE AND CHOP AHEAD

Certain vegetables lend themselves to advance chopping – carrots, cabbage, broccoli, cauliflower, capsicum, pumpkin and sweet potato. Keep each vegetable separate. Avoid prepping soft and moist vegetables (onion and garlic) and herbs as they will oxidise.

COOK DOUBLE

Look for recipes such that lend themselves to being doubled and eaten over multiple nights, such as soups, stews and curries. Not all food will last all week in the fridge so aim to also use the freezer for storage.

CONTAINERS

Purchase good quality BPA-free plastic or glass containers for food storage. Use plastic for the freezer as glass containers can expand and crack. And don't forget to label them!

EQUIPMENT

Take advantage of a mandoline, V-slicer, food processor or Thermomix, if you have one, to assist with the prep.

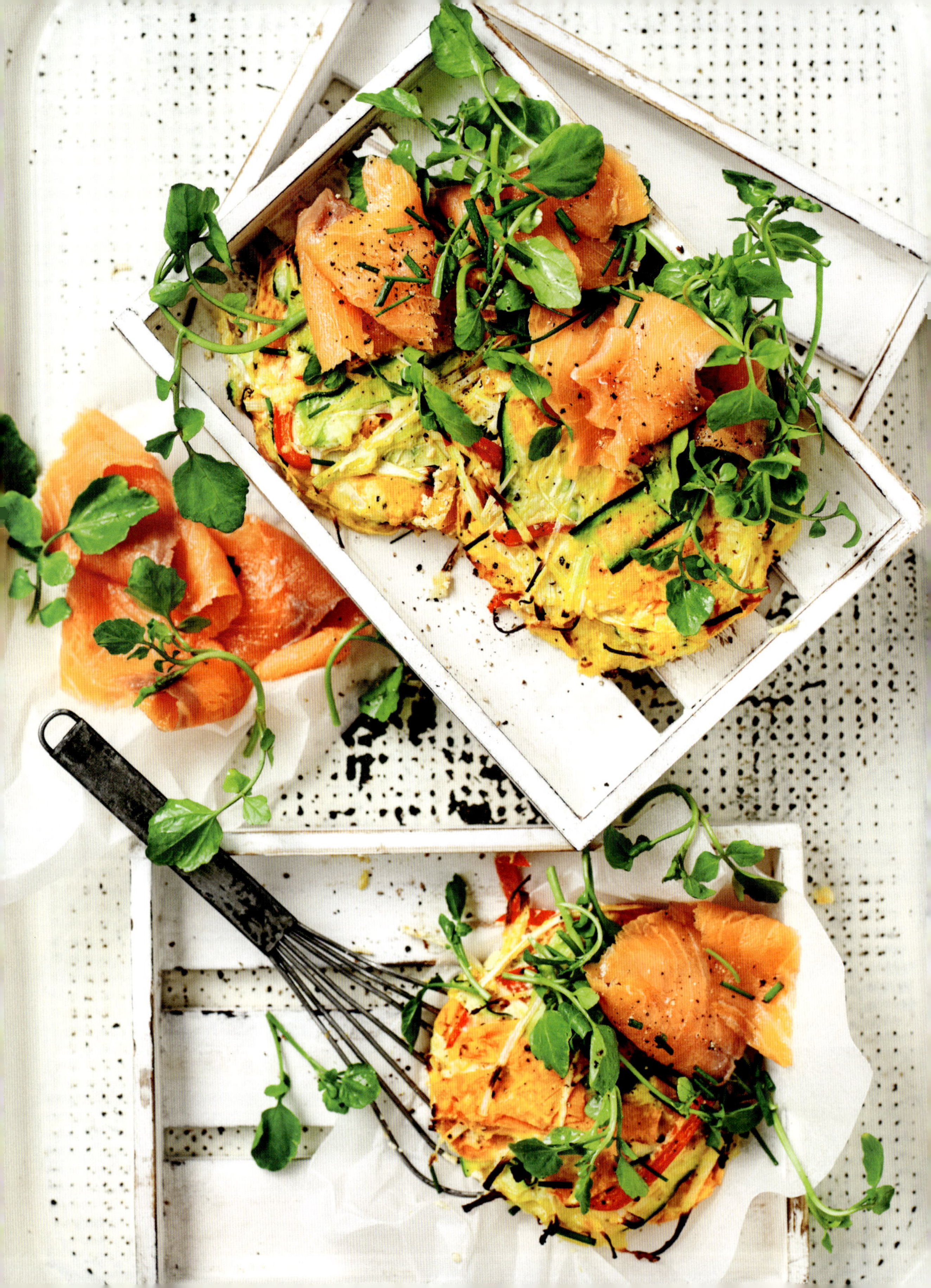

VEGIE RÖSTI WITH SMOKED SALMON & WATERCRESS

PREP + COOK TIME *40 MINUTES*
SERVES *4*

- **1 medium zucchini (120g)**
- **1 large carrot (180g)**
- **1 medium leek (350g), cut into julienne**
- **1 large red capsicum (350g), seeded, sliced thinly**
- **1 cup (240g) ricotta**
- **½ cup (50g) grated mozzarella**
- **1 extra-large egg (60g), beaten lightly**
- **50g watercress sprigs**
- **1 tsp red wine vinegar**
- **1 tbsp extra virgin olive oil**
- **200g sliced smoked salmon**

1 Preheat oven to 180°C. Line a large oven tray with baking paper.

2 Using a vegetable peeler, peel zucchini and carrot into long thin ribbons. Combine zucchini and carrot with leek, capsicum, ricotta, mozzarella and egg in a large bowl; season well.

3 Press a quarter of the vegie mixture into a 10cm round cutter on the tray. Remove cutter; repeat with remaining vegie mixture to make 4 rounds in total. Bake rounds for 25 minutes or until browned lightly and crisp.

4 Meanwhile, combine watercress, vinegar and oil in a medium bowl; season to taste.

5 Transfer vegie rösti to a platter; top evenly with smoked salmon and watercress mixture. Season to taste.

PREP IT Portion cooked vegie rösti into containers; refrigerate for up to 4 days. Serve topped with smoked salmon and watercress salad.

NUTRITION PER SERVE *19G TOTAL FAT (7G SATURATED FAT); 1351KJ (323 CAL); 9G CARBOHYDRATE; 25G PROTEIN; 5G FIBRE*

CORIANDER & LIME TOFU WITH MEXICAN SLAW

PREP + COOK TIME *35 MINUTES (+ REFRIGERATION)*
SERVES *4*

- **1 bunch coriander**
- **⅓ cup (80ml) lime juice**
- **2 long red chillies, seeded, chopped finely**
- **¼ cup (60ml) extra virgin olive oil**
- **300g firm tofu, cut into 8 long slices**
- **1 large avocado (320g)**
- **½ clove garlic, crushed**
- **1 medium carrot (120g), julienned**
- **1 medium purple carrot (120g), julienned**
- **2 cups (160g) shredded savoy cabbage**
- **4 radishes (140g), trimmed, sliced thinly**
- **8 soft wholegrain tortillas, warmed**
- **lime wedges, to serve**

1 Wash coriander well to remove all dirt from stems. Finely chop coriander roots and stems; reserve leaves for slaw.

2 Combine chopped coriander, 2 tablespoons of the lime juice, half the chilli and 1 tablespoon oil in a shallow bowl. Add tofu; toss to coat well. Cover; refrigerate for at least 2 hours or overnight.

3 To make guacamole, coarsely mash avocado in a small bowl; stir in garlic, 1 tablespoon of the lime juice and remaining chilli. Season to taste.

4 To make dressing, combine 1 tablespoon oil and remaining lime juice in a jug; season to taste.

5 Place carrots, cabbage, radish and reserved coriander leaves in a large bowl with the dressing; toss to combine.

6 Drain tofu well, reserving marinade. Heat remaining oil in a medium frying pan over medium-high heat. Cook tofu for 1 minute each side or until golden.

7 Serve tortillas topped with slaw, guacamole and tofu; drizzle with reserved marinade and serve with lime wedges.

TIP If you're short on time, you could use a packet of purchased coleslaw mix.

NUTRITION PER SERVING *42G TOTAL FAT (7.9G SATURATED FAT); 3373KJ (806 CAL); 74.4G CARBOHYDRATE; 23.6G PROTEIN; 18.8G FIBRE*

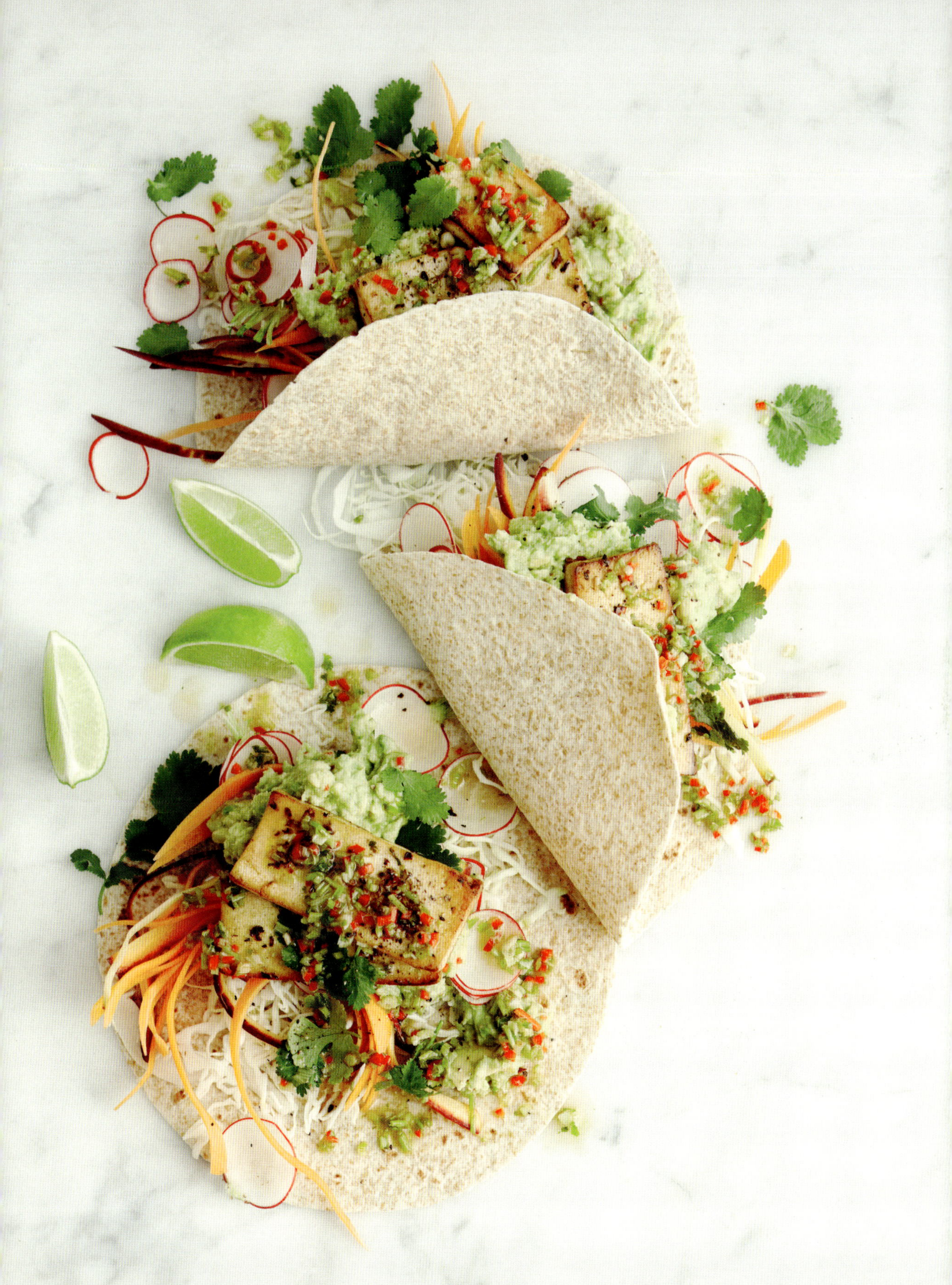

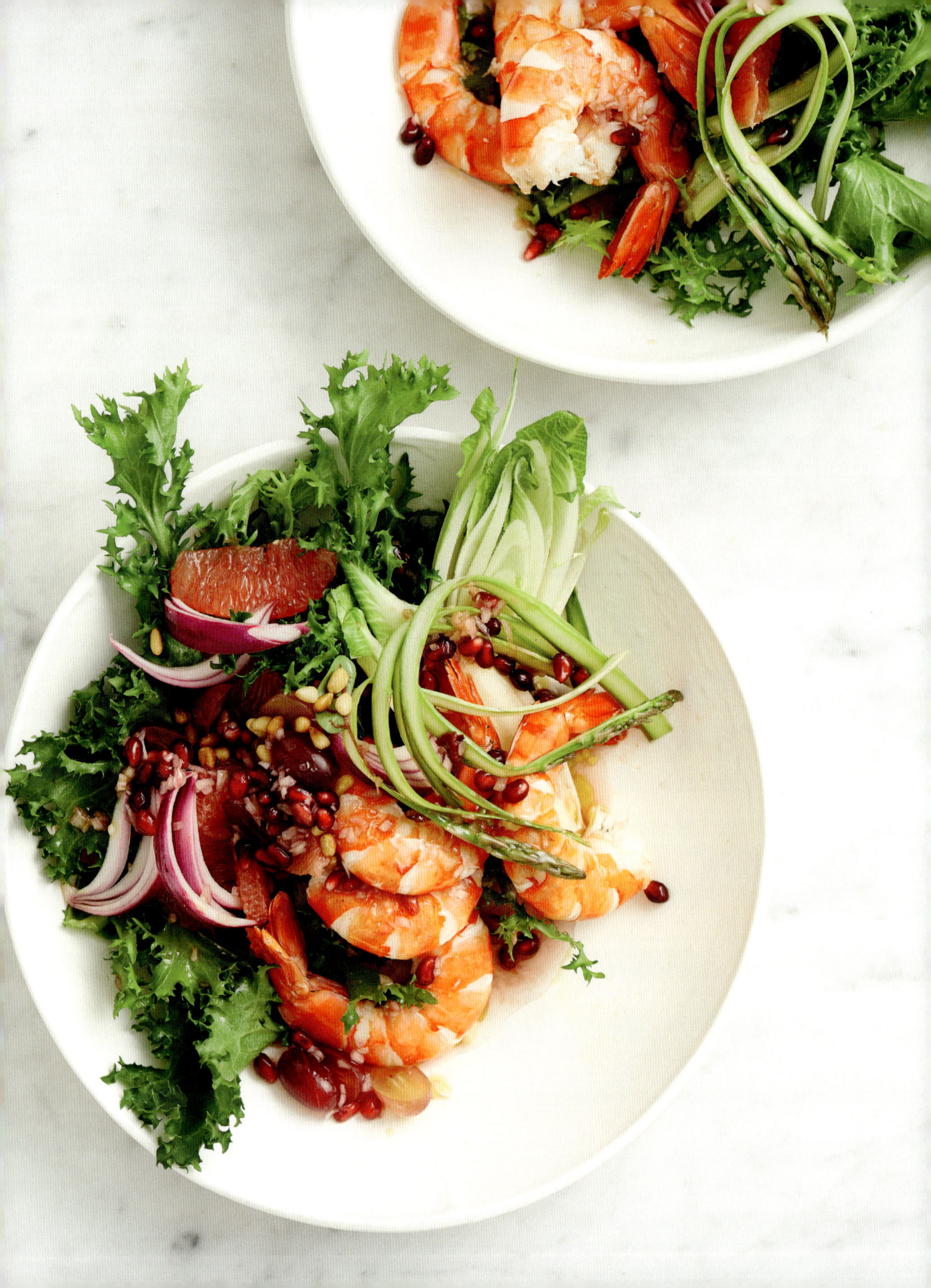

GRAPEFRUIT & PRAWN SALAD

PREP + COOK TIME *30 MINUTES*
SERVES 4

⅓ cup (50g) pine nuts

24 medium cooked prawns (840g)

400g asparagus, trimmed

300g curly endive lettuce, leaves separated

2 small witlof (200g), halved

400g seedless red grapes, halved

1 small red onion (100g), sliced thinly

GRAPEFRUIT DRESSING

2 large red grapefruits (1kg)

75g pomegranate seeds (arils) (see tip)

2 eschalots, chopped finely

¼ cup (60ml) extra virgin olive oil

1½ tbsp raspberry vinegar

1 To make the grapefruit dressing, segment the grapefruit by cutting off the rind thickly so no white pith remains. Cut between membranes, over a bowl to catch any juice, releasing segments; reserve segments in another small bowl. Squeeze juice from the membrane into bowl with juices; you will need 2 tablespoons juice. Whisk juice, pomegranate seeds, eschalots, oil and vinegar to combine; season.

2 Toast pine nuts in a frying pan over medium heat for 5 minutes or until lightly browned. Remove from pan; cool.

3 Peel and devein prawns, leaving the tails intact.

4 Using a mandoline or V-slicer, cut asparagus into thin ribbons.

5 To serve, combine endive, witlof, asparagus, grapes, onion and the reserved grapefruit; drizzle with half the dressing. Top with prawns, pine nuts and remaining dressing. Season to taste.

TIP Pomegranate seeds (arils) are available in packs from greengrocers and larger supermarkets.

NUTRITION PER SERVING *24G TOTAL FAT (2.9G SATURATED FAT); 1880KJ (449 CAL); 30.3G CARBOHYDRATE; 21.9G PROTEIN; 12.4G FIBRE*

BUTTER CHICKEN SALAD WITH GARLIC NAAN

PREP + COOK TIME *40 MINUTES (+ REFRIGERATION)*
SERVES *4*

- **3 x 200g chicken breast fillets**
- **½ cup (125ml) butter chicken simmer sauce**
- **2 tbsp extra virgin olive oil**
- **2 garlic naan breads (250g)**
- **2 tbsp red wine vinegar**
- **1 tbsp caster sugar**
- **2 tsp sea salt flakes**
- **2 small Lebanese cucumbers (200g)**
- **2 medium carrots (240g), cut into ribbons**
- **1 tsp cumin seeds, toasted**
- **½ cup (140g) Greek yoghurt**
- **1 tbsp lime pickle**
- **250g vine-ripened yellow cherry tomatoes, halved**
- **250g microwave brown and wild rice**
- **1 butter lettuce (195g), leaves separated**

1 Place chicken, simmer sauce and half the oil in a medium bowl; toss to coat well. Cover; refrigerate for 30 minutes.

2 Brush naan with remaining oil. Cook naan on heated grill plate (or grill pan) for 3 minutes each side or until crisp. Remove from grill plate; cut into wedges.

3 Remove chicken from marinade; reserve marinade. Cook chicken on lightly oiled heated grill plate over medium-high heat for 6 minutes each side or until cooked through. Transfer to a plate; keep warm.

4 Combine vinegar, sugar and salt in a bowl; transfer 1 tablespoon of the vinegar mixture to a small bowl. Cut 1 cucumber in half lengthways; remove seeds with a spoon. Cut halves lengthways again into long wedges; cut lengths into quarters. Add to vinegar mixture in large bowl with carrot and cumin seeds; toss. Grate remaining cucumber; add to reserved vinegar mixture in small bowl with yoghurt, stir to combine. Season to taste.

5 Combine lime pickle and tomatoes in a bowl.

6 Heat reserved chicken marinade in a small saucepan over medium heat until mixture boils. Remove from heat.

7 Heat rice according to packet directions.

8 Arrange lettuce on a large platter or bowl; top with sliced chicken and rice, then drizzle with hot marinade. Layer with pickled cucumber mixture and tomato mixture. Serve with cucumber yoghurt and naan bread.

NUTRITION PER SERVING *36.5G TOTAL FAT (9.5G SATURATED FAT); 3655KJ (874 CAL); 94.4G CARBOHYDRATE; 32.1G PROTEIN; 8.9G FIBRE*

TIP Use chicken thigh fillets instead of chicken breast fillets, if preferred.

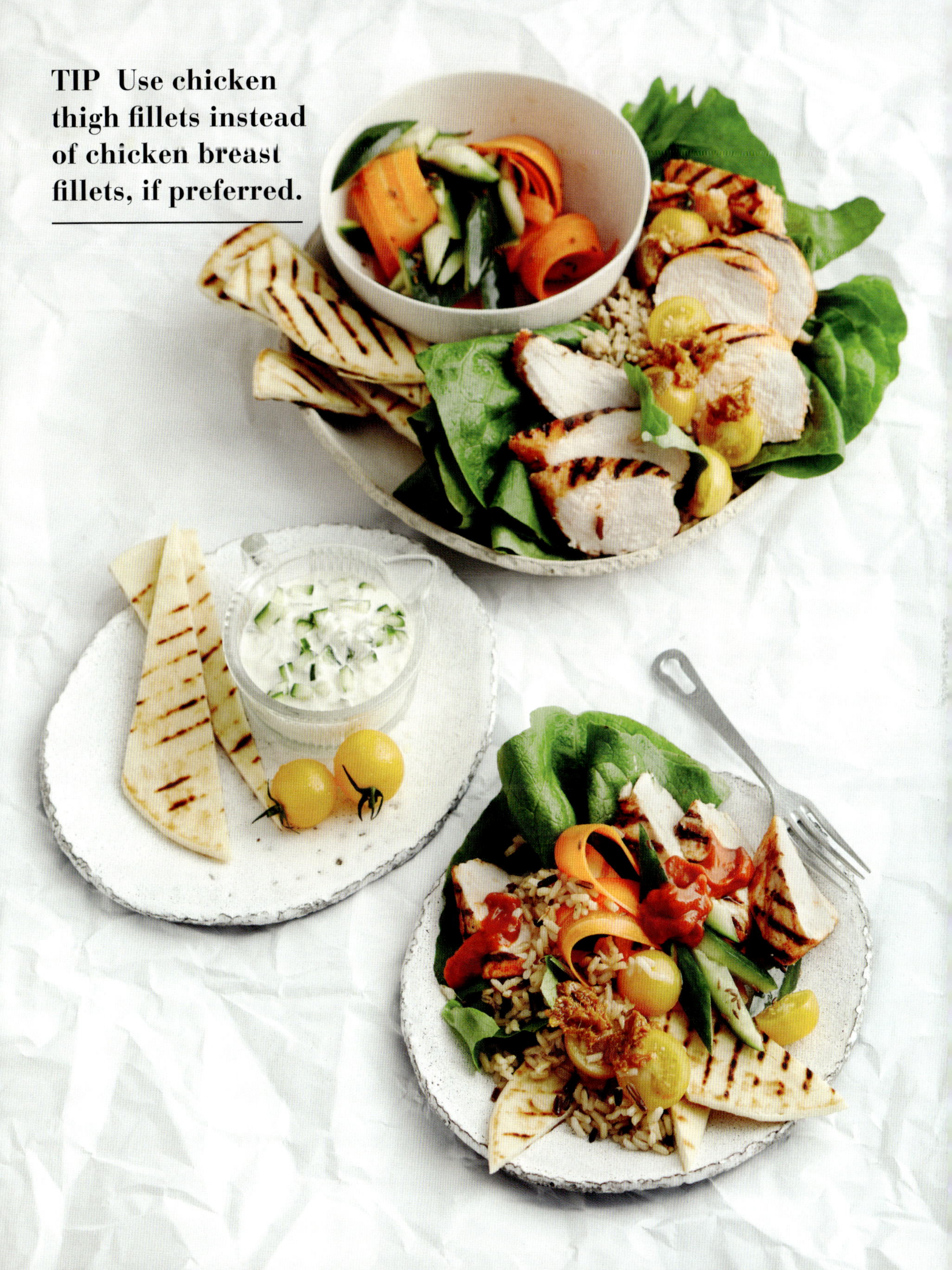

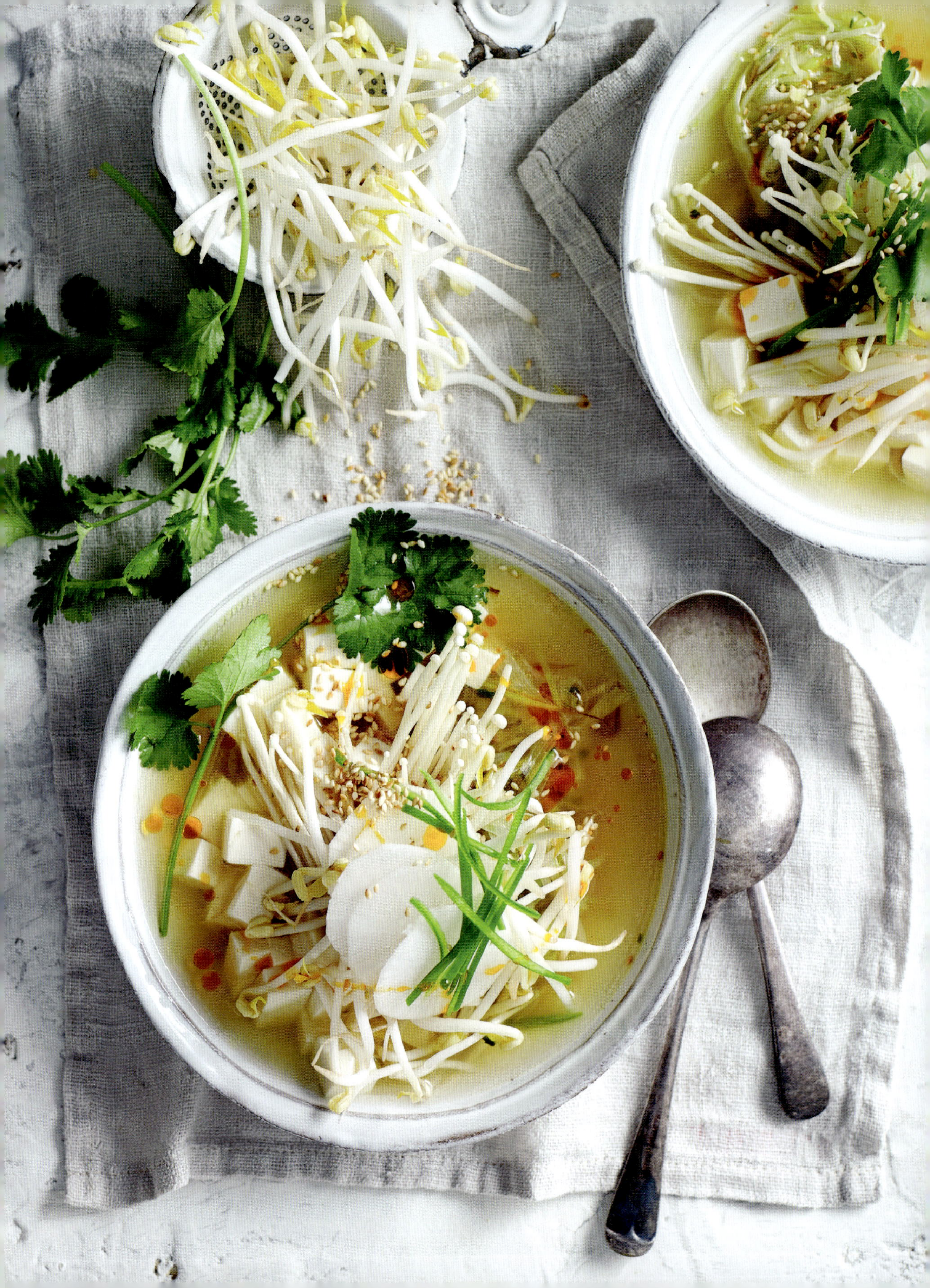

MISO, TOFU & GINGER BROTH

PREP + COOK TIME *25 MINUTES*
SERVES *4*

1 bunch coriander

1 tbsp extra virgin olive oil

1 tbsp finely grated fresh ginger

1 medium leek (350g), chopped finely

2 cups (500ml) vegetable stock

¼ cup (60g) dashi miso paste (see tip)

1 small daikon (400g), peeled, sliced thinly

600g silken tofu, drained, cut into 2cm cubes

150g bean sprouts, trimmed

180g enoki mushrooms, trimmed

1 long green chilli, seeds removed, cut into long thin strips

1 tbsp toasted sesame seeds

1 tsp chilli oil

1 Wash coriander well to remove all dirt from stems. Finely chop coriander roots and stems; reserve leaves for serving.

2 Heat olive oil in a large saucepan over medium heat; cook chopped coriander roots and stems with ginger and leek, stirring, for 3 minutes or until leek is soft. Add stock, miso and 1 litre (4 cups) water; bring to the boil. Add daikon; cook for 10 minutes or until daikon is just tender. Season to taste. Transfer daikon with a slotted spoon to a small plate lined with paper towel.

3 Divide tofu, sprouts and mushrooms between bowls. Ladle soup into bowls; top with daikon, green chilli, sesame seeds, chilli oil and reserved coriander leaves.

TIP Dashi miso paste is available from Asian supermarkets.

DO-AHEAD Soup is best made close to serving.

NUTRITION PER SERVING *13.2G TOTAL FAT (1.9G SATURATED FAT); 1073KJ (256 CAL); 13.5G CARBOHYDRATE; 15.3G PROTEIN; 11.1G FIBRE*

TURKEY LETTUCE CUPS

PREP + COOK TIME *25 MINUTES*
SERVES *4*

- **2 tbsp extra virgin olive oil**
- **1 medium onion (100g), sliced thinly**
- **4cm piece fresh ginger, peeled, grated finely**
- **3 cloves garlic, crushed**
- **500g turkey mince**
- **2 green onions, sliced thinly**
- **2 tbsp soy sauce**
- **1 tbsp lime juice**
- **1 cup coriander leaves**
- **1 cup Thai basil leaves**
- **250g bean sprouts**
- **8 small iceberg lettuce leaves, separated into cups**
- **2 medium carrots (240g), julienned**
- **1 long red chilli, seeded, sliced thinly lengthways**
- **chopped roasted peanuts and lime wedges, to serve**

1 Heat a large wok over medium heat. Add oil and onion; stir-fry for 2 minutes or until onion is softened but not coloured. Add ginger and garlic; stir-fry for 1 minute. Remove onion mixture from wok.

2 Stir-fry turkey in wok, breaking up any clumps, for 5 minutes or until turkey is cooked through. Return onion mixture to wok with green onion, soy sauce and lime juice; stir-fry for 2 minutes or until well combined.

3 Combine herbs and bean sprouts in a medium bowl.

4 Divide turkey mixture among lettuce cups; top with carrot, chilli and herb mixture. Sprinkle with peanuts and serve with lime wedges.

NUTRITION PER SERVING *27.9G TOTAL FAT (7.9G SATURATED FAT); 1704KJ (407 CAL); 9.8G CARBOHYDRATE; 26.7G PROTEIN; 6.3G FIBRE*

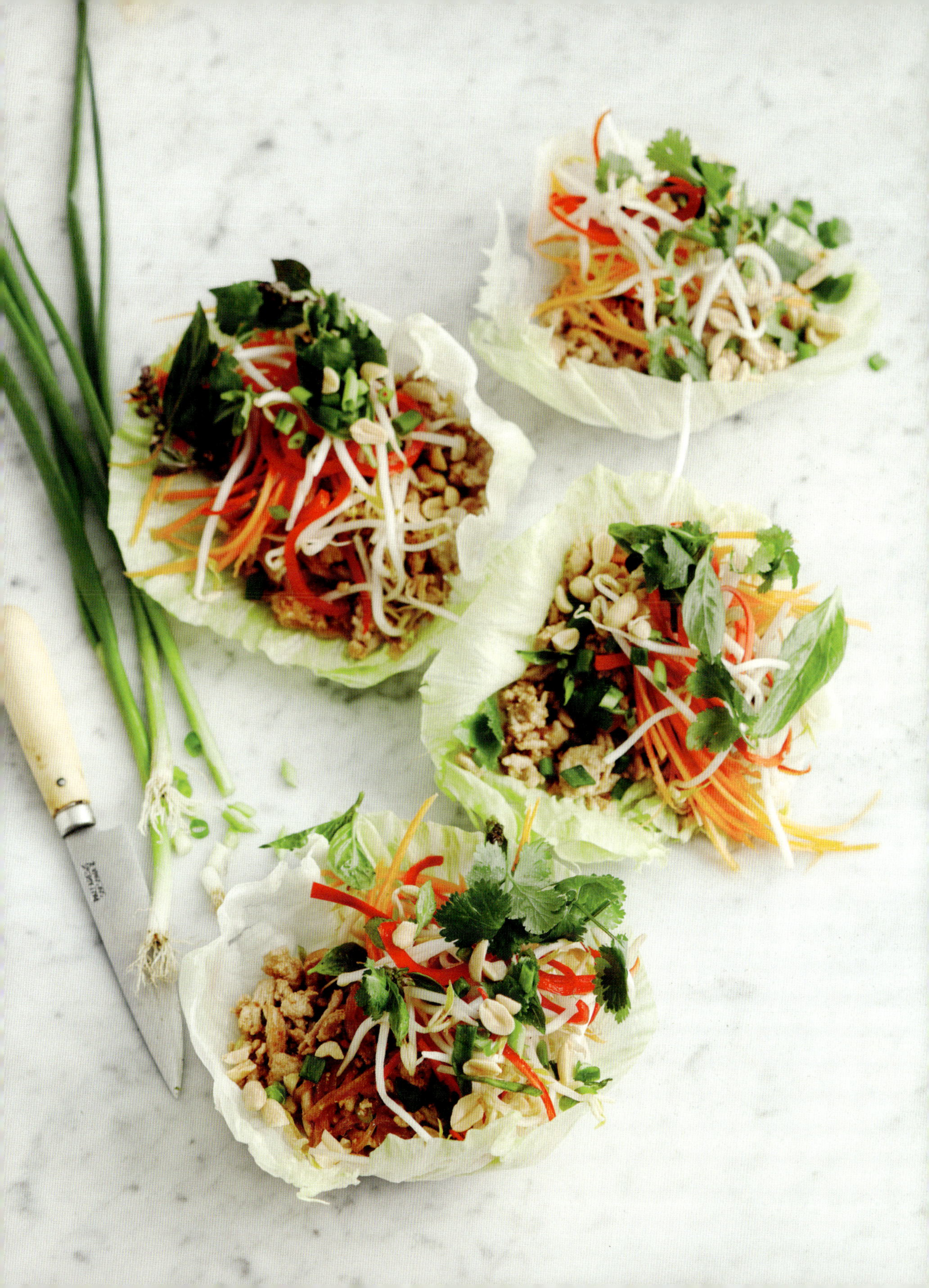

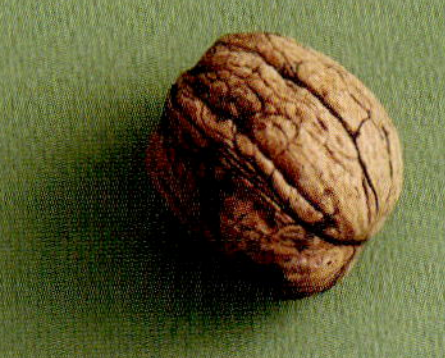

MAINS

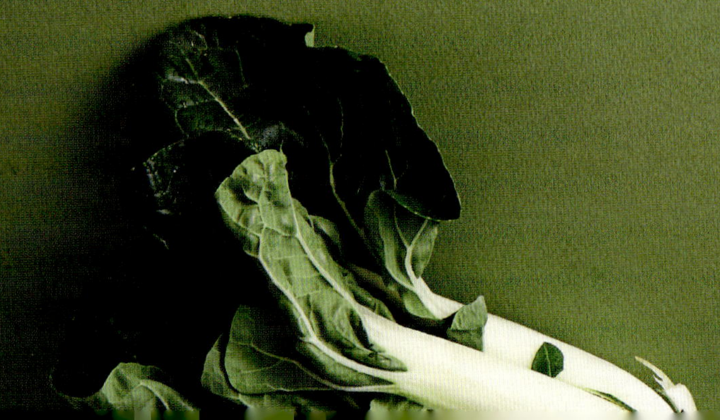

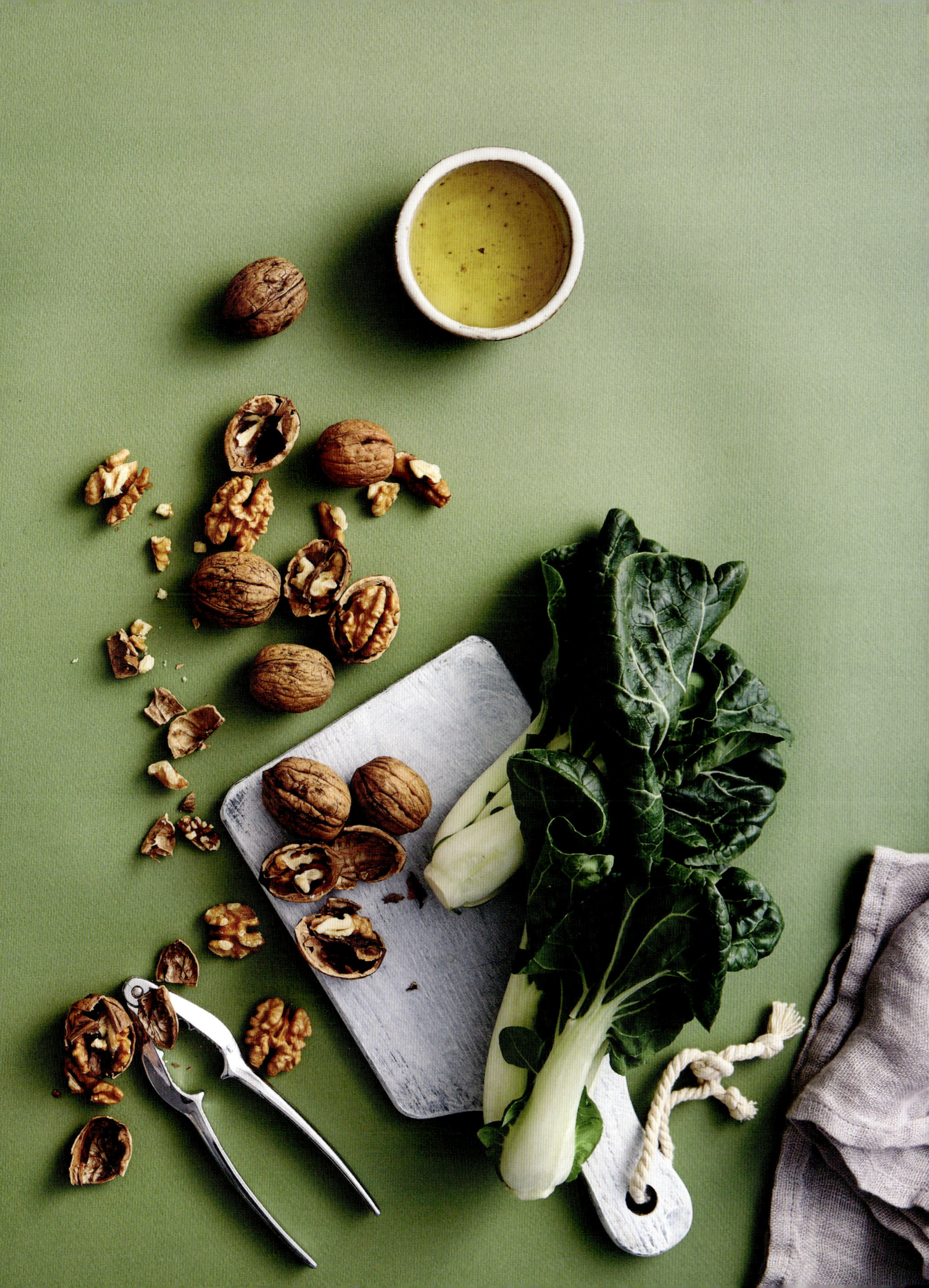

BROCCOLI SOUP WITH CRISPY QUINOA

PREP + COOK TIME *40 MINUTES*
SERVES *4*

- **1 tbsp olive oil**
- **1 medium leek (350g), sliced thinly**
- **2 stalks celery (300g), trimmed, chopped finely**
- **2 cloves garlic, crushed**
- **1 large head broccoli (400g), cut into florets**
- **2 medium zucchini (240g), chopped**
- **1 large potato (300g), peeled, chopped**
- **2¼ cups (560ml) vegetable stock**
- **⅓ cup (95g) Greek yoghurt**
- **2 slices soy and linseed bread (140g), halved, toasted**

CRISPY QUINOA

- **½ cup (100g) white quinoa, rinsed well**
- **2 tbsp olive oil**
- **2 tbsp sunflower seeds**
- **2 tbsp chopped roasted almonds**
- **1 tsp chilli flakes**
- **2 cloves garlic, crushed**
- **2 tbsp finely chopped flat-leaf parsley**

1 Heat oil in a heavy-based saucepan over medium-high heat. Add leek and celery; cook, stirring, for 3 minutes or until softened. Add garlic; cook for 1 minute.

2 Add broccoli, zucchini, potato, stock and 2¾ cups (680ml) water to pan; bring to the boil. Reduce heat to low-medium; simmer for 10 minutes or until vegetables are tender. Remove from heat; cool.

3 Meanwhile, to make crispy quinoa, cook quinoa according to packet directions. Heat oil in a frying pan over medium heat. Add quinoa, sunflower seeds, almonds and chilli flakes; cook, stirring, for 10 minutes or until quinoa browns lightly. Add garlic and parsley; cook, stirring, for 1 minute or until fragrant. Transfer to a plate; it will crisp as it cools.

4 Blend or process broccoli mixture until smooth. Season to taste.

5 Divide soup among four bowls; top each with 1 tablespoon of the yoghurt and season with pepper. Sprinkle with crispy quinoa and serve with toast.

PREP IT Portion soup and crispy quinoa, separately, into airtight containers. Store soup in the fridge and quinoa at room temperature for up to 4 days. Reheat the soup just before serving and top with crispy quinoa.

NUTRITION PER SERVING *26.7G TOTAL FAT (3.6G SATURATED FAT); 2145KJ (512 CAL); 41.9G CARBOHYDRATE; 19.4G PROTEIN; 13.2G FIBRE*

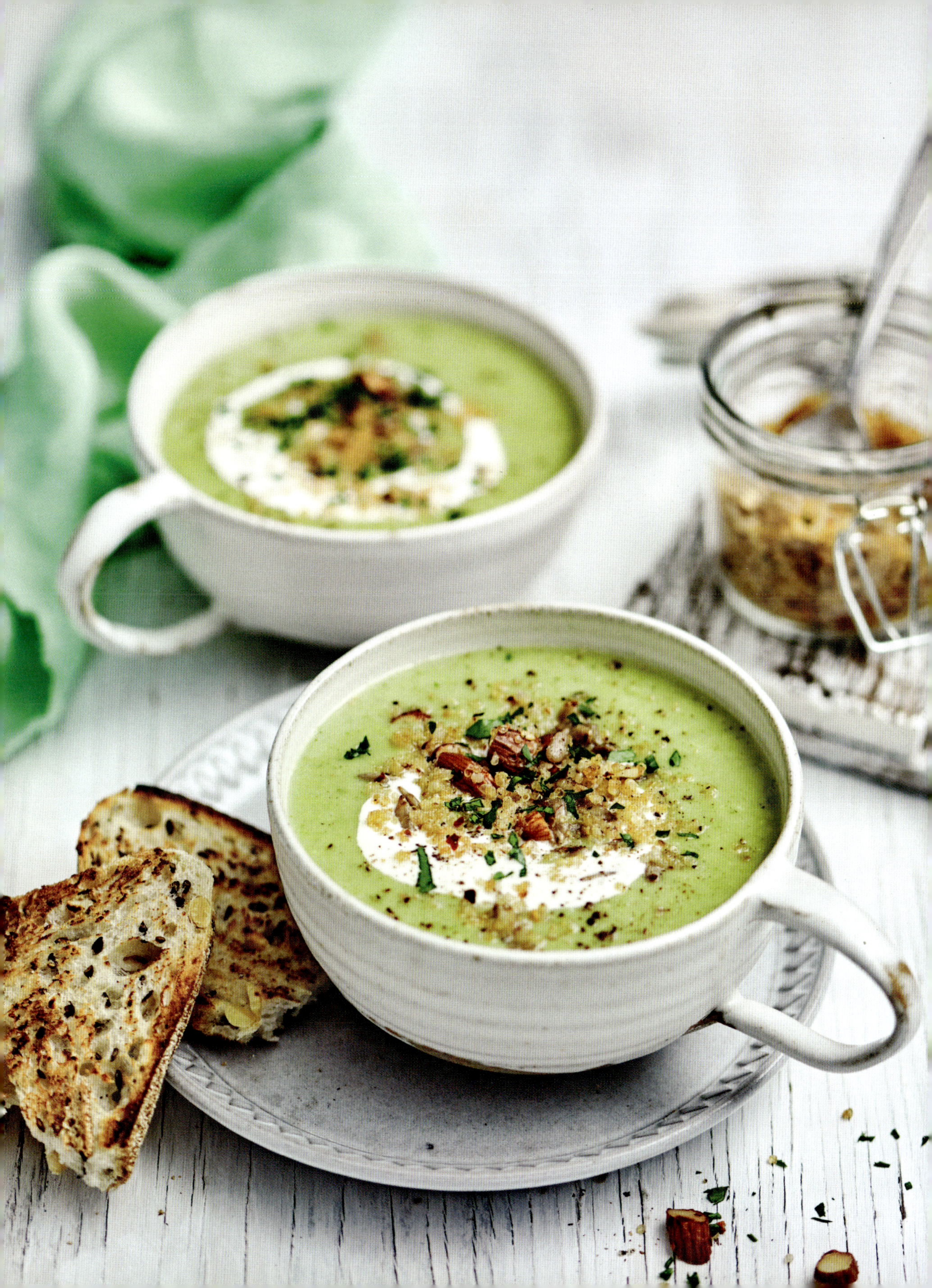

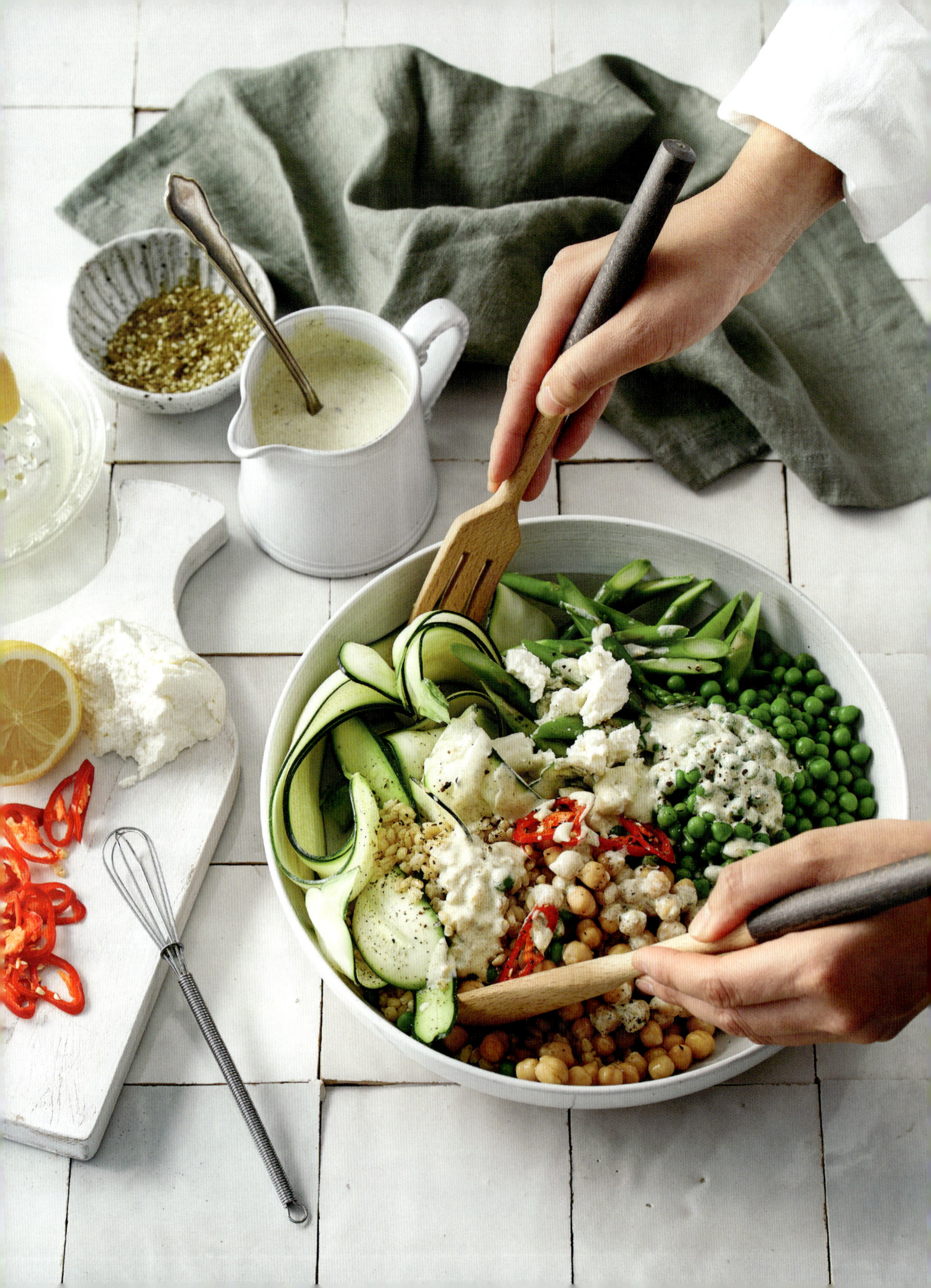

WARM BARLEY, CHICKPEA, ASPARAGUS & PEA SALAD

PREP + COOK TIME *45 MINUTES*
SERVES 4

¾ cup (150g) pearl barley
1 bunch asparagus (170g), cut into thirds on the diagonal
¾ cup (90g) frozen peas
¾ cup (190g) Greek yoghurt
2 tbsp lemon juice
1 tsp finely grated lemon rind
1 tbsp za'atar, plus extra to serve
½ tsp ground cumin
2 tbsp extra virgin olive oil
2 medium zucchini (240g), peeled into ribbons
¼ cup mint leaves, chopped finely
¼ cup dill, chopped
400g can chickpeas, drained, rinsed
1 long red chilli, sliced finely
250g firm ricotta, crumbled

1 Cook barley in a saucepan of boiling water for 35 minutes or until tender. Drain.

2 Place asparagus and peas in heatproof bowl; cover with boiling water. Stand for 1 minute. Drain well.

3 To make the dressing, whisk yoghurt, lemon juice and rind, za'atar, cumin, olive oil and 2 tablespoons water in a bowl until combined. Season to taste.

4 Place barley, asparagus and peas in a medium bowl with zucchini, herbs, chickpeas, chilli and dressing; toss to combine. Season to taste. Serve topped with ricotta and extra za'atar.

TIP Barley is a nutritious grain, commonly used in soups and stews. Hulled barley, the least processed form of barley, is high in fibre. Pearl barley has had the husk removed then been steamed and polished so that only the "pearl" of the original grain remains, much the same as white rice.

NUTRITION PER SERVING *21.5G TOTAL FAT (7.6G SATURATED FAT); 1998KJ (478 CAL); 43.3 CARBOHYDRATE; 20G PROTEIN; 12.6 FIBRE*

ZUCCHINI, SPINACH & SWEET POTATO FRITTATA

PREP + COOK TIME *1 HOUR*
SERVES 4

1 tbsp extra virgin olive oil

1 medium leek (350g), sliced thinly

2 cloves garlic, crushed

200g baby spinach leaves

6 extra-large eggs (60g each), beaten lightly

1 small orange sweet potato (250g), grated coarsely

1 cup (180g) cooked brown rice (see tip)

⅓ cup basil leaves, chopped coarsely

100g firm ricotta, crumbled

30g finely grated parmesan

2 large zucchini (300g), sliced thinly lengthways into ribbons

olive oil spray

60g rocket leaves

2 tbsp small basil leaves, extra

1 Preheat oven to 180°C. Grease a 20cm x 30cm slice pan; line base with baking paper.

2 Heat 2 teaspoons of the oil in a frying pan over medium heat; cook leek and garlic, stirring, for 5 minutes or until softened. Add spinach, stir until wilted; cool.

3 Blend or process spinach mixture and egg until spinach is finely chopped but not pureed. Pour into a large bowl; stir in sweet potato, rice, basil, ricotta and ¼ cup of the parmesan. Season.

4 Pour mixture into pan, top with overlapping zucchini slices, placing them lengthways; press in lightly. Spray lightly with oil; sprinkle with remaining parmesan.

5 Bake for 30 minutes or until egg mixture is set. Stand in pan for 5 minutes to cool, before cutting evenly into eight pieces.

6 Drizzle remaining oil over rocket leaves. Serve two pieces of frittata each, topped with rocket and extra basil leaves.

TIP You will need to cook about ⅓ cup raw low-GI doongara brown rice for the quantity of cooked cooled rice needed for the recipe. Doongara rice, grown exclusively in Australia, is a naturally low-GI rice variety available from major supermarkets.

PREP IT Portion the frittata into containers; refrigerate for up to 4 days. Serve reheated or at room temperature.

NUTRITION PER SERVING *16.5G TOTAL FAT (4.6G SATURATED FAT); 1452KJ (346 CAL); 26.6G CARBOHYDRATE; 19.7G PROTEIN; 6.1G FIBRE*

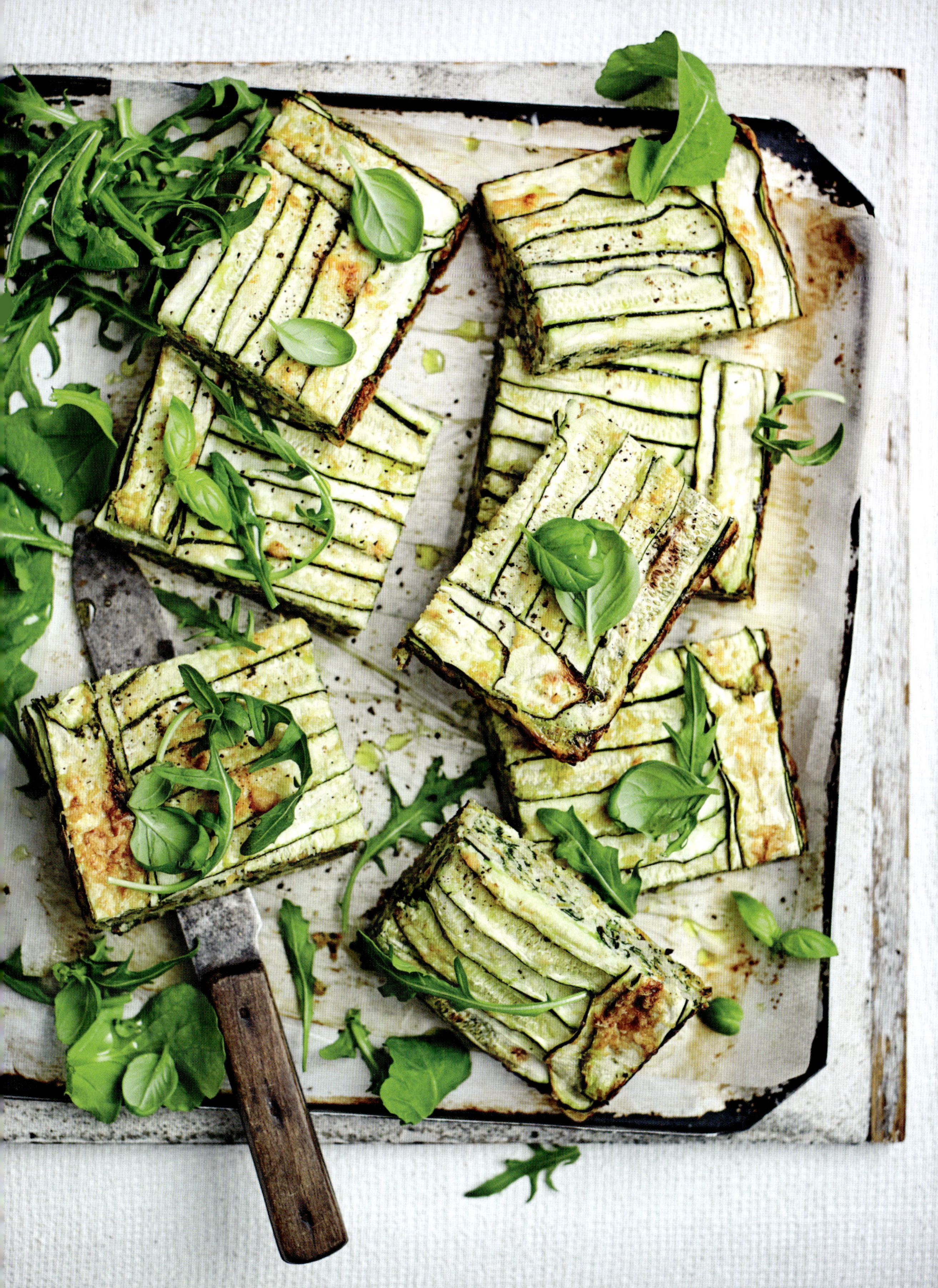

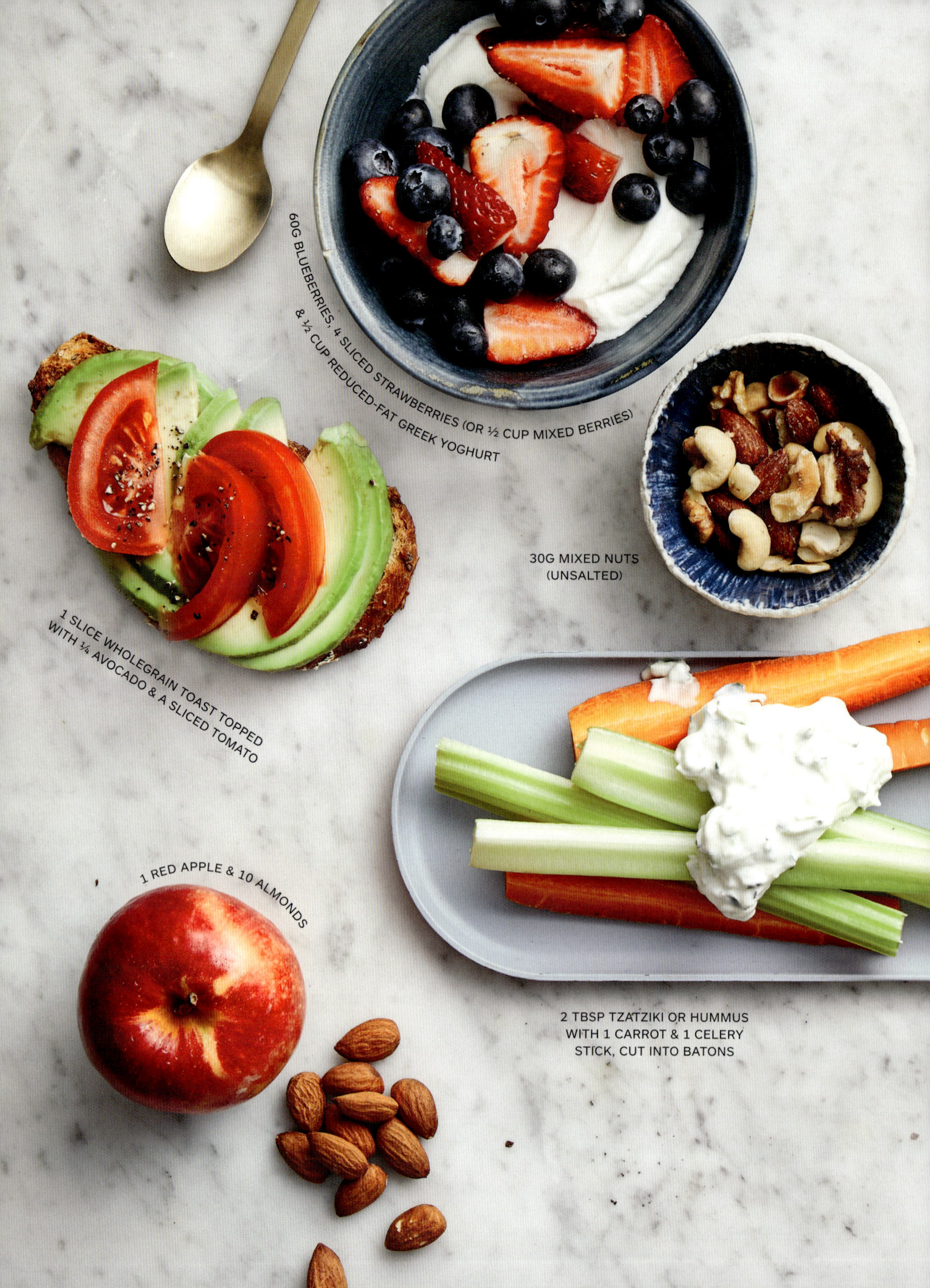
60G BLUEBERRIES, 4 SLICED STRAWBERRIES (OR ½ CUP MIXED BERRIES)
& ½ CUP REDUCED-FAT GREEK YOGHURT
30G MIXED NUTS
(UNSALTED)
1 SLICE WHOLEGRAIN TOAST TOPPED
WITH ¼ AVOCADO & A SLICED TOMATO
1 RED APPLE & 10 ALMONDS
2 TBSP TZATZIKI OR HUMMUS
WITH 1 CARROT & 1 CELERY
STICK, CUT INTO BATONS

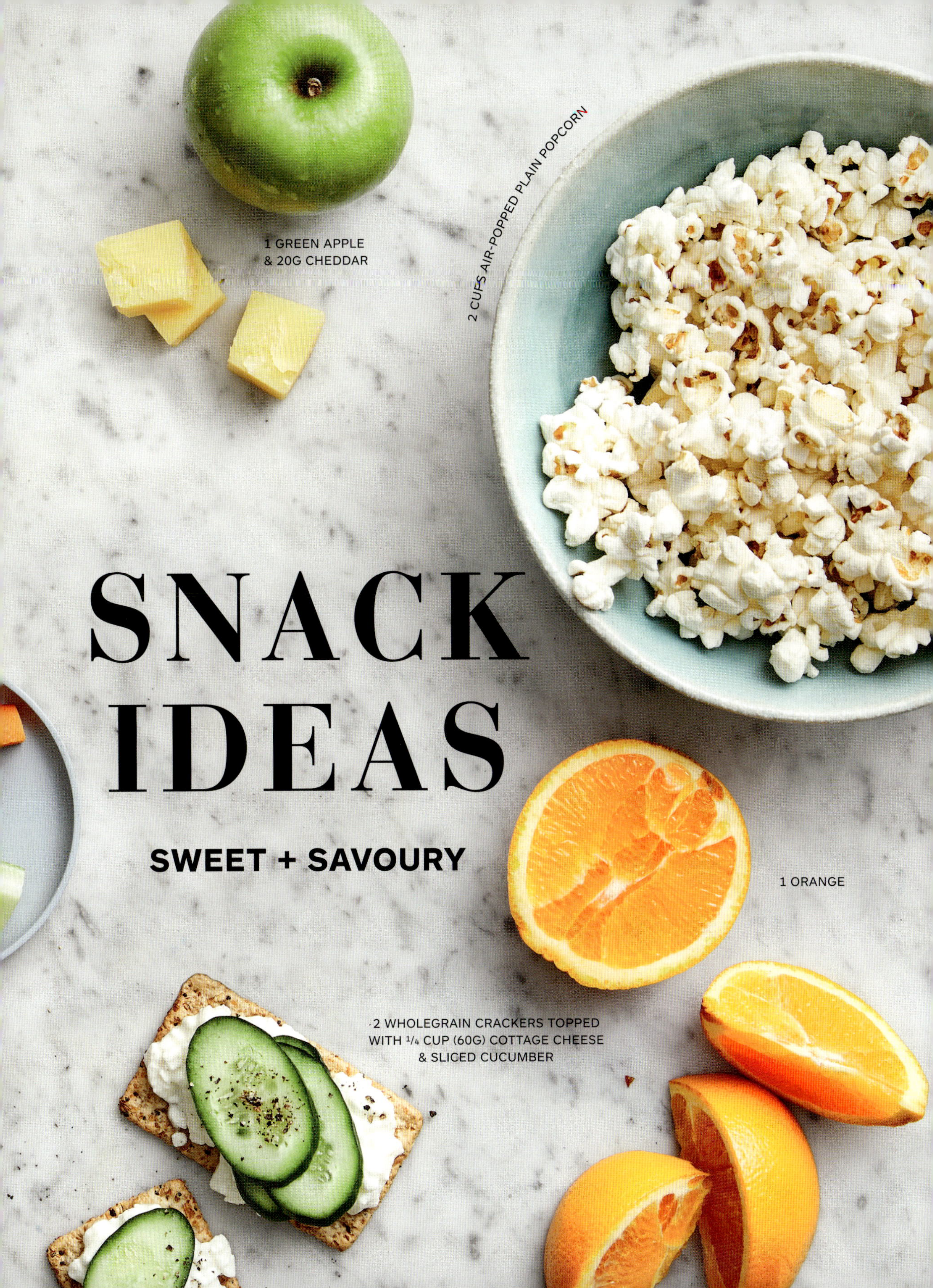
SNACK IDEAS
SWEET + SAVOURY
1 GREEN APPLE & 20G CHEDDAR
2 CUPS AIR-POPPED PLAIN POPCORN
1 ORANGE
2 WHOLEGRAIN CRACKERS TOPPED WITH 1/4 CUP (60G) COTTAGE CHEESE & SLICED CUCUMBER

ROASTED SUMMER VEG COUSCOUS BOWL

PREP + COOK TIME *35 MINUTES*
SERVES *2*

2 small zucchini (180g), halved lengthways

200g firm tofu, patted dry, cut into 10 slices

¼ cup (50g) drained, rinsed, canned chickpeas

250g cherry truss tomatoes

2 cloves garlic, sliced thinly

2 tsp Moroccan seasoning

170g asparagus, trimmed, halved lengthways

200g yellow patty-pan squash

¼ cup (50g) wholemeal couscous

¼ cup (20g) quinoa flakes

1 tsp grated lemon rind

60g baby rocket leaves

1 tbsp lemon juice

½ cup basil leaves

1 Preheat oven to 220°C. Line two large oven trays with baking paper.

2 Place zucchini, tofu, chickpeas and half the tomatoes on one tray, then add garlic and Moroccan seasoning; toss to coat. Turn zucchini, cut-side down; roast mixture for 10 minutes. Place asparagus, squash and remaining tomatoes on second tray; roast in oven with zucchini mixture for 8 minutes or until asparagus is just tender and zucchini is browned.

3 Meanwhile, combine couscous, quinoa and lemon rind in a small heatproof bowl. Add ½ cup (125ml) boiling water; cover immediately. Stand for 5 minutes or until liquid is absorbed. Fluff with a fork; season to taste.

4 Divide rocket between two bowls; top with couscous mixture, tofu and roasted vegetables. Drizzle with lemon juice and top with basil; serve.

NUTRITION PER SERVING *9.6G TOTAL FAT (1.2G SATURATED FAT); 1559KJ (372 CAL); 38.1G CARBOHYDRATE; 25.8G PROTEIN; 13.8G FIBRE*

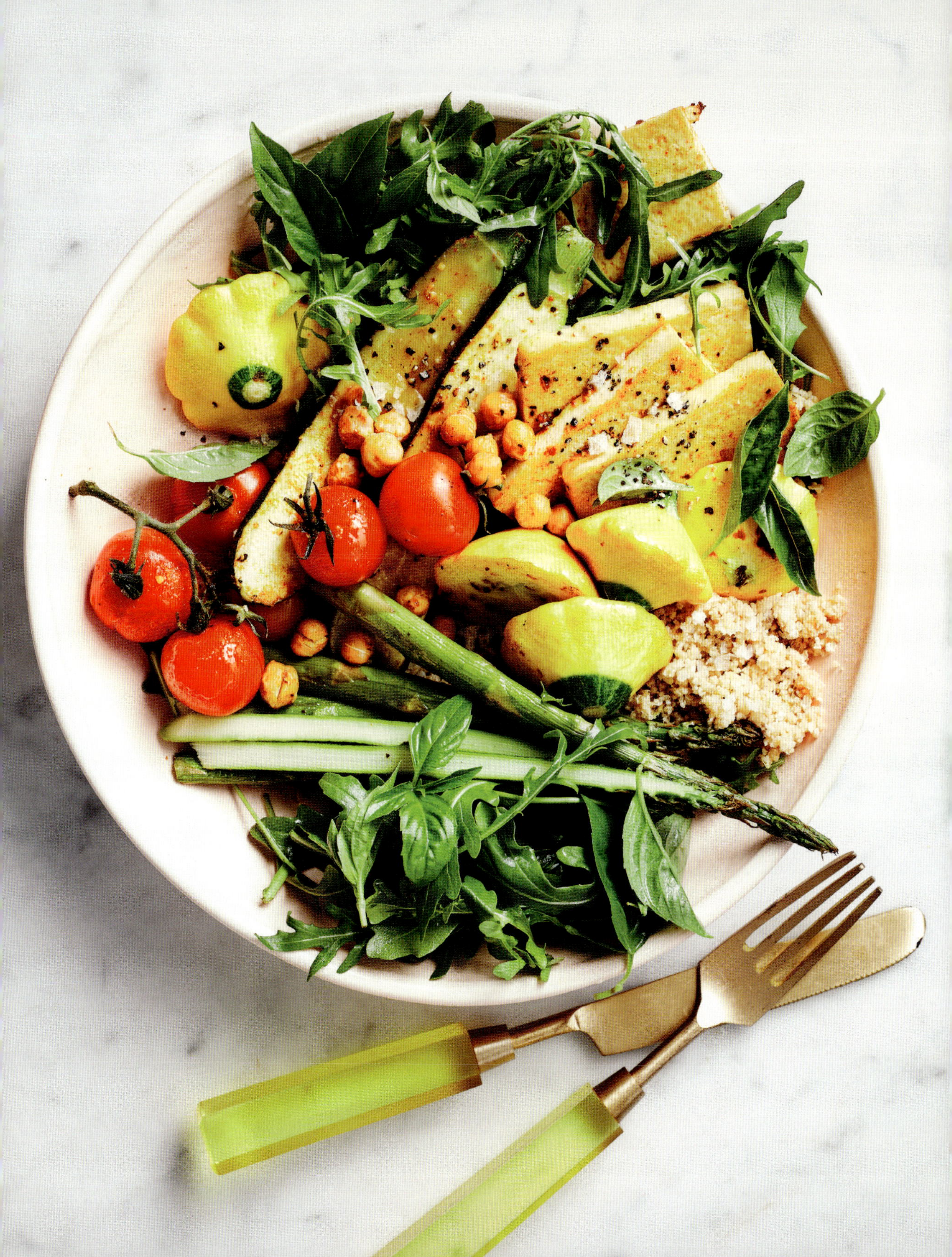

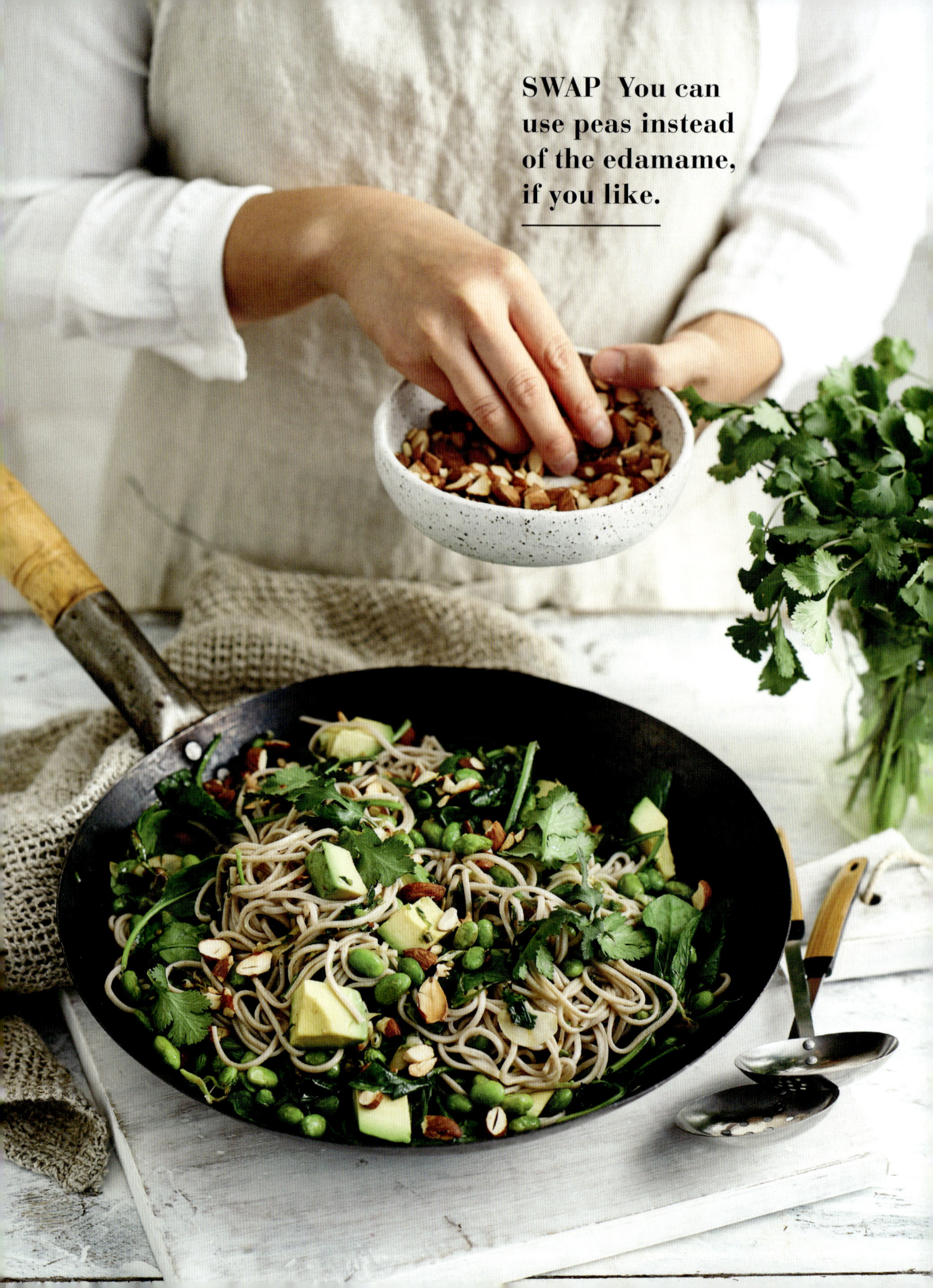

SWAP You can use peas instead of the edamame, if you like.

EDAMAME, AVOCADO & SPINACH SOBA NOODLES

PREP + COOK TIME *30 MINUTES*
SERVES *4*

- **4 green tea bags**
- **250g buckwheat soba noodles**
- **2 cups (300g) frozen shelled edamame, thawed**
- **1 tbsp sesame oil**
- **2 green onions, sliced thinly**
- **3 cloves garlic, sliced thinly**
- **1 long green chilli, chopped finely**
- **120g baby spinach leaves**
- **1 cup coriander leaves, chopped coarsely**
- **¼ cup (60ml) lime juice**
- **2 medium avocados (500g), chopped coarsely**
- **½ cup (80g) almonds, roasted, chopped**

1 Bring 3 litres (12 cups) water to the boil in a large saucepan. Turn off the heat. Add tea bags; steep for 10 minutes. Discard tea bags.

2 Fill a large bowl with cold water. Return tea water to the boil; add soba noodles, then cook for 5 minutes or until tender. Drain, reserving ½ cup (125ml) cooking liquid. Working quickly, refresh noodles in the cold water; drain. Cover until ready to serve.

3 Pat thawed edamame dry with paper towel. Heat oil in a wok or large frying pan over high heat. Add green onion, garlic and chilli; cook, stirring frequently, for 1 minute or until fragrant. Add edamame; cook, stirring occasionally, for 2 minutes or until edamame are blistered slightly.

4 Add noodles to wok with spinach, half the coriander, the lime juice and reserved cooking liquid; cook, tossing continuously, for 2 minutes or until well combined and spinach has wilted.

5 Serve noodle mixture topped with avocado, remaining coriander and the almonds.

TIPS Make sure to buy unsalted edamame. Seed the chilli if you prefer less heat.

NUTRITION PER SERVING *35.1G TOTAL FAT (4.5G SATURATED FAT); 2689KJ (643 CAL); 52.4G CARBOHYDRATE; 20.4G PROTEIN; 21G FIBRE*

EGGPLANT BOLOGNESE BAKE

PREP + COOK TIME *1 HOUR 45 MINUTES*
SERVES *6*

2 medium eggplant (600g)
200g baby spinach leaves
¾ cup (180g) ricotta
1 extra-large egg white (from 60g egg)
½ cup (50g) coarsely grated mozzarella
⅓ cup (25g) coarsely grated parmesan
50g baby rocket leaves

BOLOGNESE SAUCE

1 tbsp olive oil
1 large onion (200g), chopped
1 small red capsicum (150g), seeded, chopped coarsely
1 small green capsicum (150g), seeded, chopped coarsely
2 cloves garlic, crushed
250g lean beef mince
1 tbsp tomato paste
½ cup (125ml) dry red wine
400g can chopped tomatoes
2 tbsp chopped basil

1 Preheat oven to 180°C.

2 To make bolognese sauce, heat oil in a medium frying pan over medium heat; cook onion, capsicums and garlic, stirring, for 5 minutes or until onion softens. Remove from pan. Increase heat to high, add beef; cook, stirring, for 5 minutes or until beef is browned all over. Return vegetables to pan with tomato paste; cook, stirring, for 3 minutes. Add wine; cook, stirring, for a further 2 minutes. Add tomatoes; bring to the boil. Reduce heat; simmer for 25 minutes or until mixture thickens slightly. Stir in basil; season to taste.

3 Meanwhile, cut eggplant into 2mm thick slices; cook eggplant slices on a heated oiled grill plate (or grill pan) until just tender.

4 Boil, steam or microwave spinach until wilted; drain. Squeeze as much liquid as possible from spinach; cool for 10 minutes. Combine spinach, ricotta and egg white in a medium bowl; season.

5 Spread 1 cup of the bolognese sauce over base of a shallow 2-litre (8-cup) ovenproof dish. Layer with half the eggplant, half the spinach mixture and another 1 cup of bolognese sauce. Repeat layering with remaining eggplant, spinach mixture and bolognese sauce. Top with mozzarella and parmesan.

6 Bake for 20 minutes or until cheeses are browned. Stand for 10 minutes. Serve with rocket leaves.

NUTRITION PER SERVING *15.8G TOTAL FAT (7.2G SATURATED FAT); 1162KJ (277 CAL); 7.2G CARBOHYDRATE; 21.6G PROTEIN; 5.4G FIBRE*

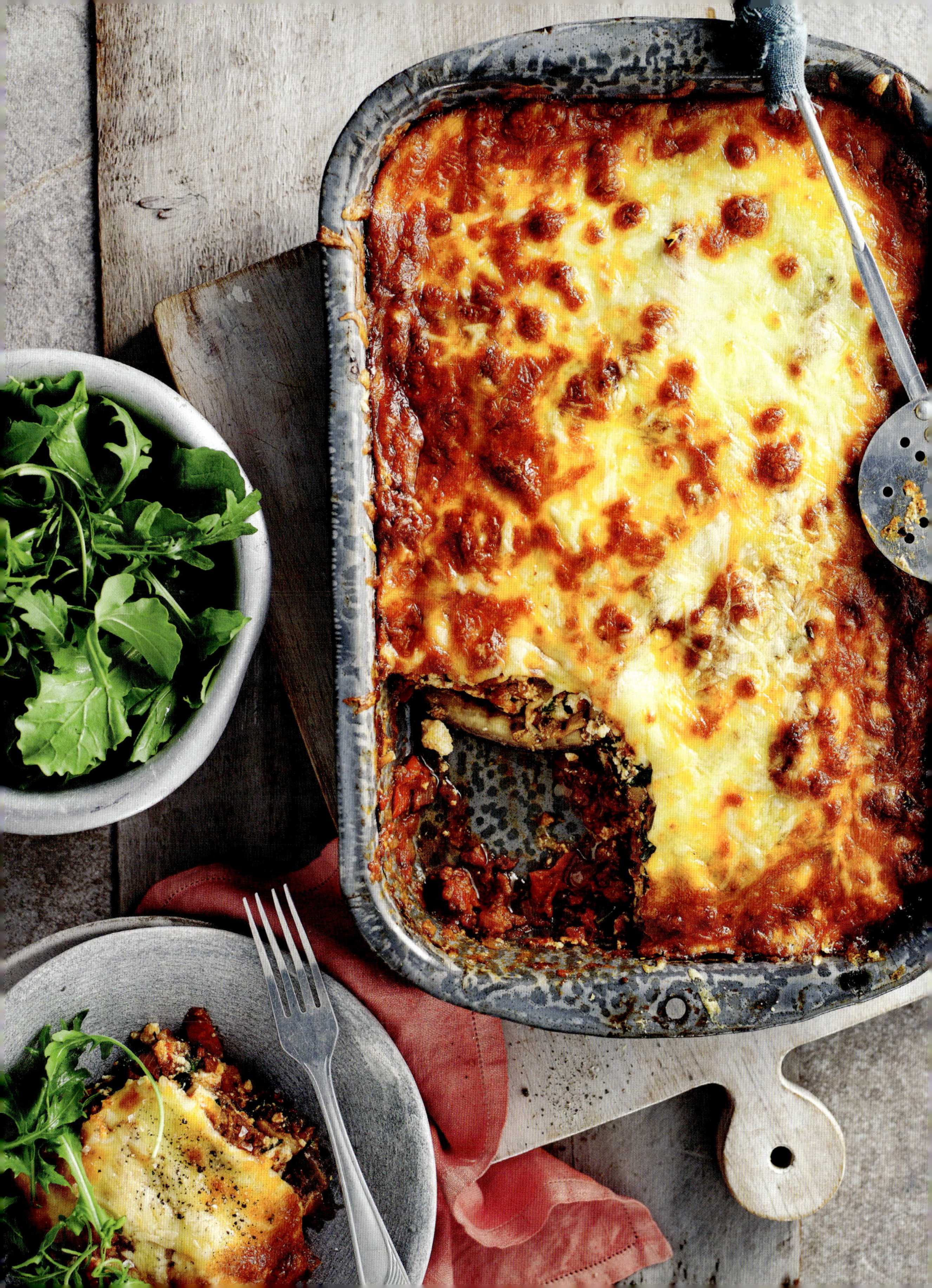

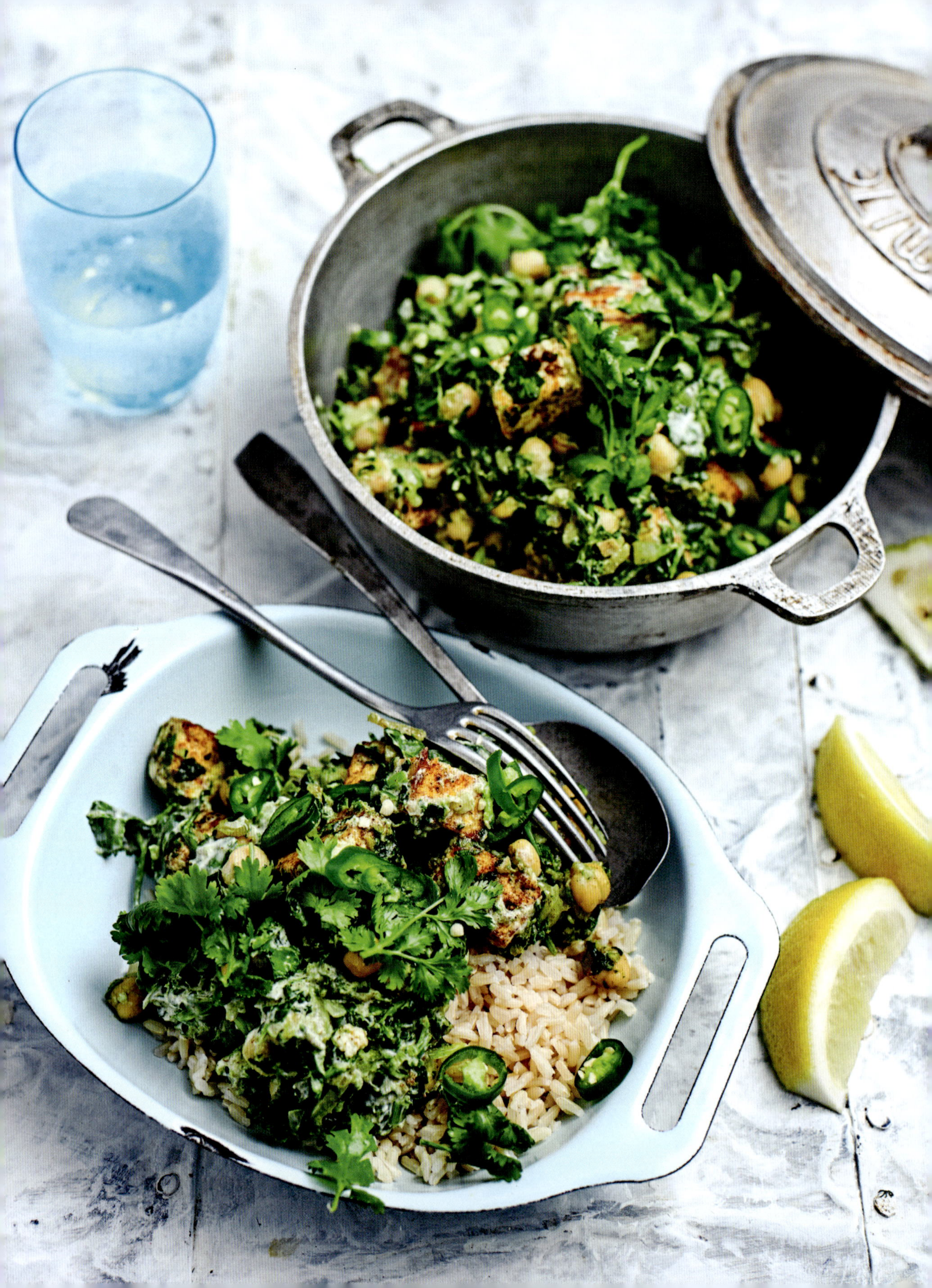

SPINACH & PANEER CURRY

PREP + COOK TIME *35 MINUTES*
SERVES *4*

¾ cup (150g) doongara low-GI brown rice (see tip)

1 bunch coriander

1 tbsp olive oil

1 medium onion (150g), sliced thinly

1 tbsp finely chopped fresh ginger

2 cloves garlic, crushed

1 long green chilli, sliced thinly

120g baby spinach leaves

200g paneer cheese, cut into 2cm cubes

1 tbsp garam masala

2 tsp ground cumin

400g can chickpeas, drained, rinsed

⅓ cup (95g) plain yoghurt

1 small lemon (65g), cut into wedges

1 Cook rice according to packet directions. Cover to keep warm. Wash coriander well to remove all dirt from stems. Pick leaves, then finely chop coriander roots and stems; reserve ½ cup leaves to serve.

2 Meanwhile, heat 2 teaspoons of the oil in a medium heavy-based frying pan over medium-high heat. Add onion; cook, stirring, for 5 minutes or until soft. Add ginger, garlic, coriander stems and roots, and half the green chilli to pan; cook for 1 minute or until fragrant. Add spinach; cook for 1 minute or until wilted.

3 Transfer spinach mixture to a food processor with coriander leaves; pulse until chopped coarsely.

4 Heat remaining oil in same pan over medium-high heat. Add paneer; cook, turning, for 2 minutes. Add spices; cook, stirring, for 1 minute or until fragrant.

5 Return spinach mixture to pan with chickpeas and yoghurt. Remove pan from heat, stir until well combined.

6 Divide rice and paneer curry among four bowls. Sprinkle with remaining chilli and reserved coriander leaves; serve with lemon wedges.

TIP Doongara rice, grown exclusively in Australia, is a naturally low-GI rice variety available from major supermarkets.

NUTRITION PER SERVING *16G TOTAL FAT (6.7G SATURATED FAT); 1735KJ (414 CAL); 43.2G CARBOHYDRATE; 19.8G PROTEIN; 8.7G FIBRE*

SWEET POTATO & ARTICHOKE SALAD WITH TAHINI-OLIVE DRESSING

PREP + COOK TIME *1 HOUR 35 MINUTES*
SERVES *4*

600g small white sweet potatoes

600g mixed fresh beans (see tips)

400g can kidney beans, drained, rinsed

360g artichoke hearts in oil, drained

TAHINI-OLIVE DRESSING

2 tbsp pitted Sicilian green olives, chopped

¼ cup (70g) tahini

⅓ cup (80ml) extra virgin olive oil

1 tsp honey

1½ tbsp red wine vinegar

1 Preheat oven to 180°C. Line an oven tray with baking paper.

2 Score sweet potatoes lengthways, making 1cm deep incisions. Place on the lined tray; roast for 50 minutes or until cooked through. Cool.

3 Meanwhile, cook fresh beans, in batches if necessary, in a large saucepan of salted boiling water for 3 minutes or until tender-crisp. Transfer to a bowl of iced water; drain.

4 To make tahini-olive dressing, process ingredients with 2 tablespoons water in a small food processor, pulsing until just combined but still coarse; season with pepper. Transfer to a small bowl.

5 Cut sweet potatoes lengthways into long wedges. Place, cut-side up, in a large shallow bowl. Top with fresh beans, kidney beans and artichokes; spoon over dressing. Season with pepper; serve.

TIPS We used a combination of snake beans, green beans and yellow beans. This creamy dressing is a great egg-free mayonnaise substitute.

NUTRITION PER SERVING *42G TOTAL FAT (15.1G SATURATED FAT); 2953KJ (706 CAL); 60.5G CARBOHYDRATE; 15.9G PROTEIN; 18.3G FIBRE*

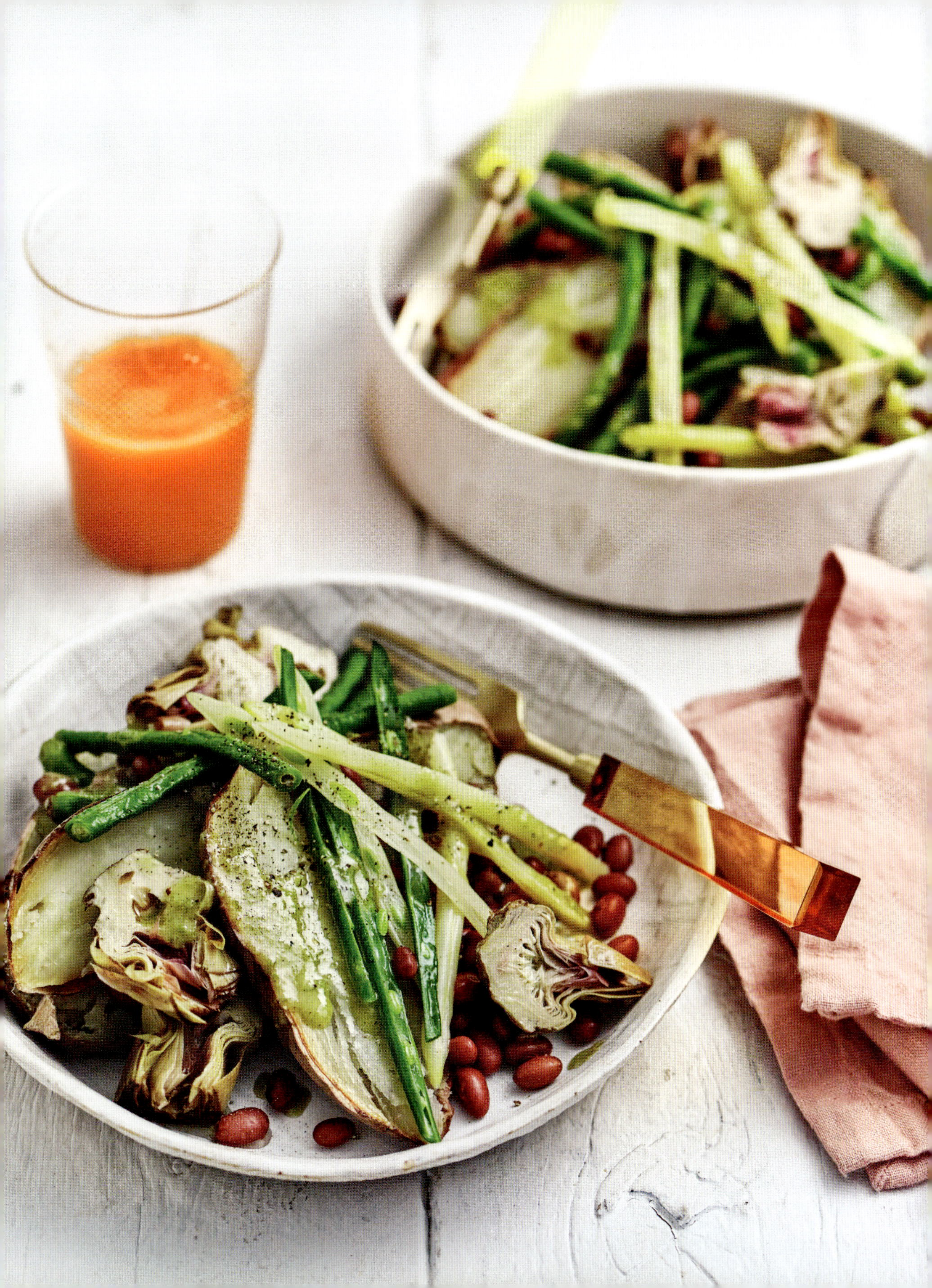

SLEEP WEIGHT CONNECTION

Not getting quality enough sleep is one of the biggest threats to our waistline. So if you're serious about your intermittent fasting, ensuring you get adequate rest is critical to keeping excess kilos off long term.

Life feels far more difficult when you haven't had much sleep. You feel lousy, have trouble concentrating, don't have as much energy, your mood might be low, you have no motivation to exercise and your food choices are all about convenience because you simply can't be bothered. Sound familiar?

When it comes to your health, a good night's sleep is just as important as regular exercise and a healthy diet. For most of us, sleeping for less than 7-8 hours can have major effects on a whole range of health risk factors including your weight.

A good night's sleep supports short-term and long-term memory and overall learning, allows our body to grow, develop and repair, strengthens the immune system, restores our energy levels, helps to reduce inflammation, supports healthy blood-sugar levels, and helps reduce our likelihood of developing depression.

When we don't get enough quality sleep, our hunger hormones can be thrown out of whack, we lose motivation to exercise, we have a larger appetite, the reward centres in our brain are more stimulated and there is reduced activity in the part of the brain in charge of decision-making and self-control. It's a cascade of events that sees people eating too much, not moving enough and making unhealthy food choices.

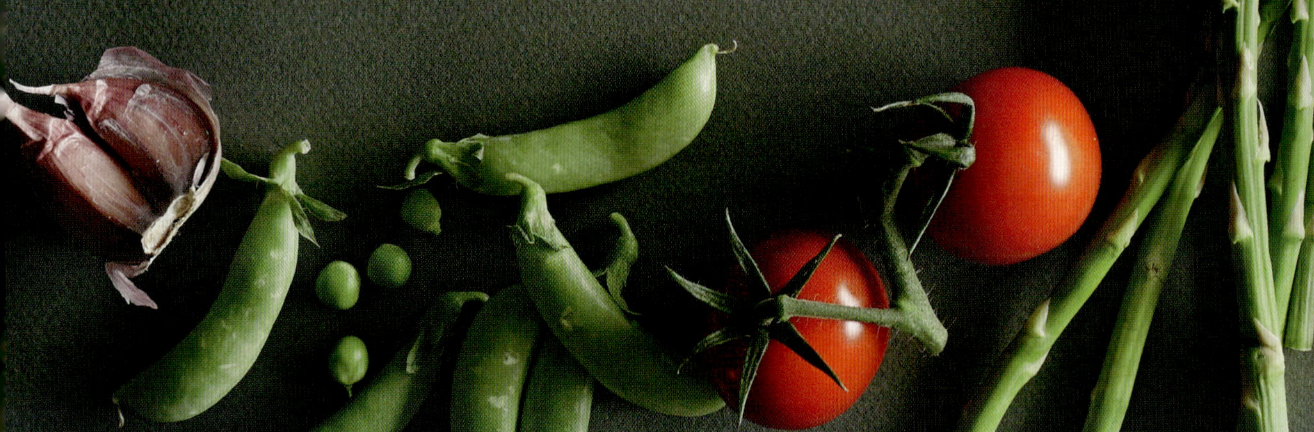

WHAT HAPPENS WHEN WE SLEEP?

There are two basic types of sleep – rapid eye movement (REM) and non-rapid eye movement. Every time you sleep, you continually cycle through four different stages – three non-REM stages and one REM stage in roughly 90-minute cycles.

The First Stage

This is the transition from an awake state to light sleep. Your heartbeat, breathing and eye movements slow and your muscles begin to relax, with occasional twitches.

The Second Stage

The is light sleep where you relax further, your body temperature drops and your eye movements stop. You spend more time in this stage than the others over the course of your sleep.

The Third Stage

This is the deep sleep required to feel refreshed in the morning. This is typically when it's the hardest to wake up, and occurs in longer periods during the first half of the night.

The Fourth Stage

This is the REM sleep which takes about 90 minutes to get to once you've started the sleep cycle. Your brain wave activity becomes closer to that seen in wakefulness, your breathing becomes faster, your heart rate and blood pressure increase, your eyes move rapidly from side to side behind closed eyelids, and your arm and leg muscles become temporarily paralysed. This is when most of your dreams happen.

TIPS & TRICKS FOR A BETTER NIGHT'S REST

If you're not sleeping too well, some simple tweaks to your evening routine, environment or coffee habit can really help. Try these out:

- Skip screen time for at least 30 minutes before bed.
- Go caffeine-free after lunch.
- Stick to a consistent routine/bedtime, on weekends too!
- Avoid alcohol before bed.
- Optimise your bedroom environment: keep it clean, cool, and free from noise and lights.
- Try relaxation techniques, such as reading, meditating, deep breathing or yoga, before bed.
- Have a warm bath or shower to relax.
- Upgrade your bed and pillow to suit your needs if you're waking up with aching muscles, bones or joints.
- Exercise during the day for a more restful sleep.

SUPER SPROUT SPAGHETTI

PREP + COOK TIME *40 MINUTES*
SERVES *4*

- **¼ cup (60ml) extra virgin olive oil**
- **500g Brussels sprouts, trimmed**
- **1 large onion (200g), chopped finely**
- **1 small carrot (70g), grated coarsely**
- **4 cloves garlic, crushed**
- **3 anchovy fillets**
- **1 tbsp finely chopped rosemary**
- **⅓ cup (95g) tomato paste**
- **2 x 400g cans diced tomatoes with Italian herbs**
- **2 x 250g packets dried pulse spaghetti (see tip)**
- **⅓ cup basil leaves**
- **finely grated parmesan, to serve**

1 Heat 1½ tablespoons of the oil in a large saucepan over high heat; cook Brussels sprouts, stirring occasionally, for 10 minutes or until lightly browned. Remove from pan.

2 Heat remaining oil in same pan over medium heat; cook onion and carrot, stirring, for 3 minutes or until softened. Add garlic, anchovies, rosemary and tomato paste; cook, stirring, for 2 minutes or until paste darkens slightly. Add canned tomatoes and ¾ cup (180ml) water; bring to the boil. Reduce heat to low; simmer, covered, for 10 minutes.

3 Meanwhile, cook pasta in a large saucepan of boiling salted water following packet directions; drain. Return pasta to pan.

4 Add sprouts and half the basil to sauce; cook, stirring, for 2 minutes or until heated through.

5 Serve pasta topped with sauce, remaining basil and the parmesan.

NUTRITION PER SERVING *22.1G TOTAL FAT (5.6G SATURATED FAT); 3133KJ (749 CAL); 87.6G CARBOHYDRATE; 39.8G PROTEIN; 21G FIBRE*

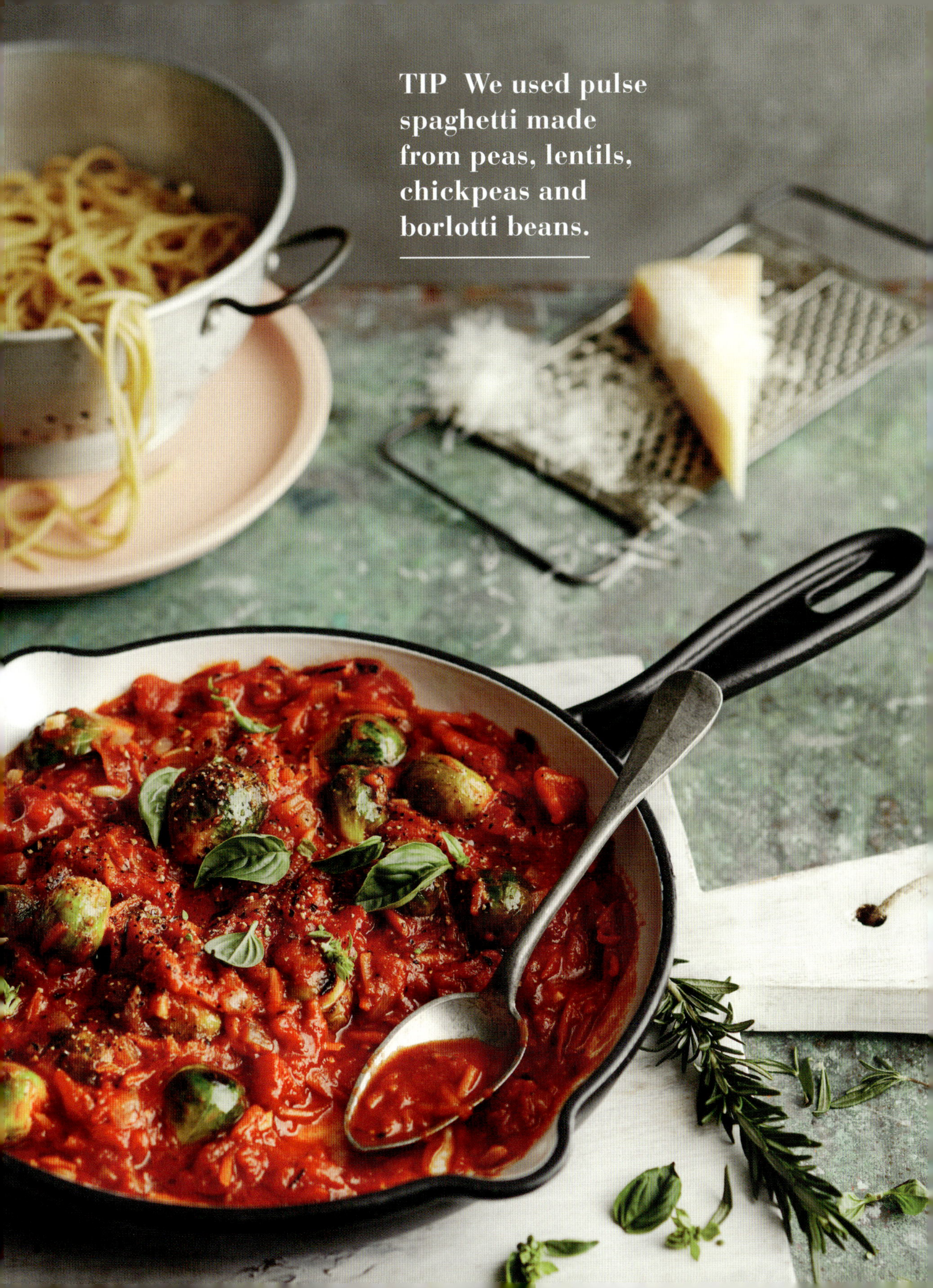

TIP We used pulse spaghetti made from peas, lentils, chickpeas and borlotti beans.

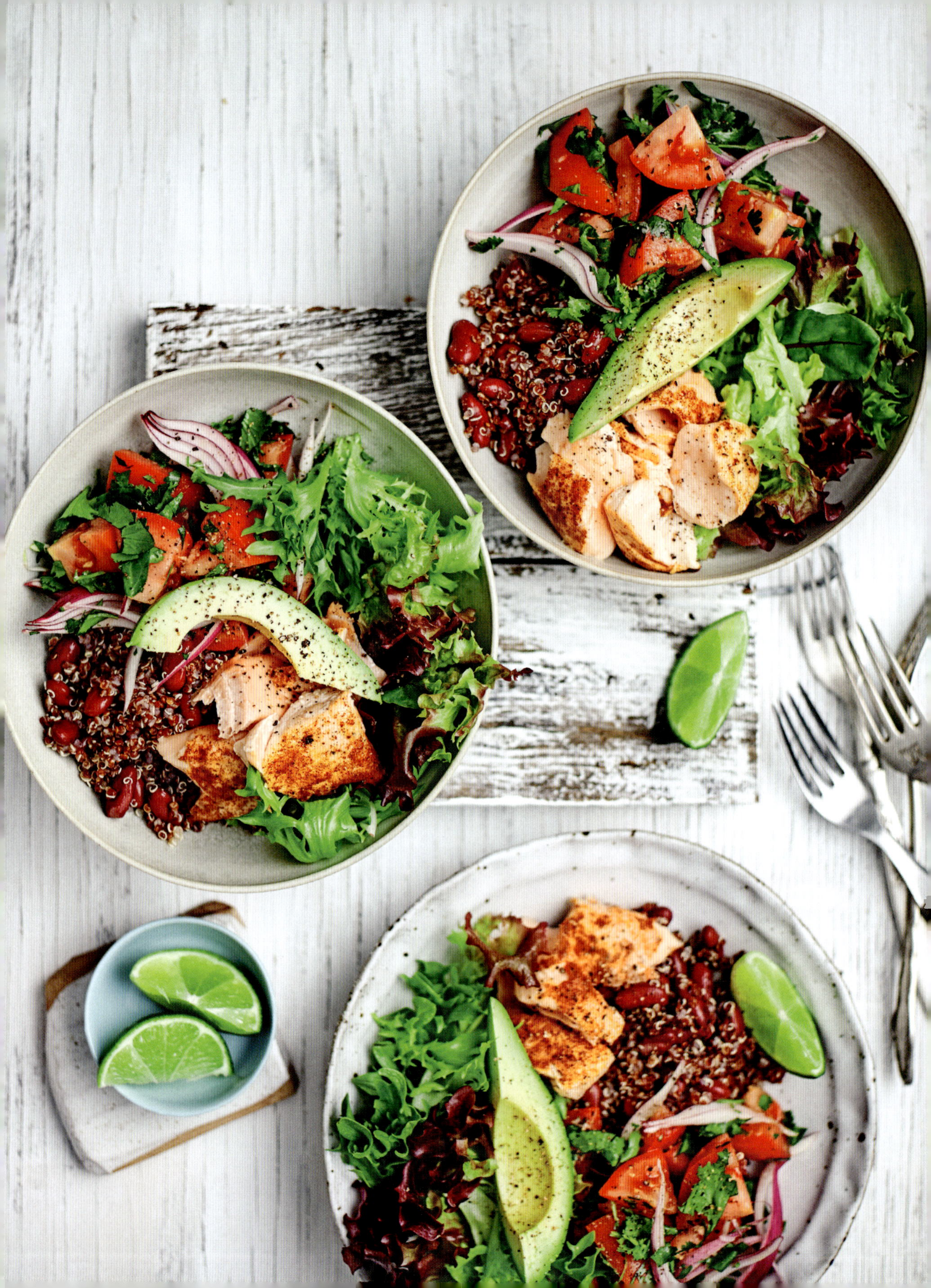

SPICY ROAST SALMON BURRITO BOWLS

PREP + COOK TIME *40 MINUTES*
SERVES *4*

½ cup (100g) red quinoa, rinsed well (see tip)
400g can kidney beans, drained, rinsed
300g skinless boneless salmon fillets
1½ tsp Mexican chilli powder
3 medium roma tomatoes (180g), chopped coarsely
1 small red onion (100g), sliced thinly
½ cup coriander leaves, chopped coarsely
2 tbsp lime juice
3 tsp olive oil
1 small clove garlic, crushed
80g mixed salad leaves
½ small avocado (100g), sliced into thin wedges
1 lime (65g), cut into wedges

1 Preheat oven to 220°C. Line a small oven tray with baking paper.

2 Place quinoa and 1 cup (250ml) water in a small saucepan; bring to the boil. Reduce heat to low; cook, covered, for 20 minutes or until water is absorbed. Remove from heat; fluff grains with a fork and stir through beans.

3 Meanwhile, place salmon fillets on oven tray; sprinkle with chilli powder. Roast salmon for 12 minutes for medium or until cooked to your liking.

4 Place tomato, onion and coriander in a bowl, season with pepper; toss to combine well.

5 Combine lime juice, oil and garlic in a small bowl. Flake salmon into large pieces. Divide quinoa mixture, tomato salad, salad leaves, avocado and salmon evenly among four bowls. Drizzle with lime dressing; season and serve with lime wedges.

TIP If you like, use white or tri-coloured quinoa instead of red quinoa.

NUTRITION PER SERVING *19.1G TOTAL FAT (4.4G SATURATED FAT); 1668KJ (398 CAL); 25.5G CARBOHYDRATE; 25.5G PROTEIN; 9.2G FIBRE*

GRILLED TURMERIC CHICKEN WITH CARROT NOODLES

PREP + COOK TIME *45 MINUTES (+ REFRIGERATION)*
SERVES *4*

4 cloves garlic, chopped

2cm piece turmeric, peeled, chopped

½ tsp rock salt

¼ cup (60ml) canned coconut milk

2 tsp fish sauce

4 x 250g chicken breast supremes (see tips)

4 medium carrots (480g)

100g dried vermicelli noodles

250g golden yellow tomatoes, halved

¼ cup (20g) fried shallots

½ cup loosely packed mint leaves

1 medium lime (90g), cut into wedges

LIME DRESSING

½ cup (125ml) lime juice

¼ cup (60ml) fish sauce

2 tbsp grated palm sugar

1½ tsp sesame oil

1 Preheat oven to 180°C.

2 Using a mortar and pestle, pound garlic, turmeric and salt to a smooth paste. Stir in coconut milk and fish sauce. Rub all over chicken; place on a plate. Cover; refrigerate for 20 minutes.

3 Heat a large grill plate (or grill pan) over medium-high heat. Cook chicken for 3 minutes each side or until dark grill marks form. Transfer chicken to a baking-paper-lined oven tray. Roast chicken for 12 minutes or until just cooked through. Cover to keep warm; stand for 5 minutes. Slice thickly.

4 Meanwhile, to make lime dressing, stir ingredients in a bowl until sugar dissolves.

5 Peel carrot into long strips with a julienne peeler or slice thinly. Place carrot and noodles in a large heatproof bowl; cover with boiling water. Stand for 1 minute; drain. Refresh carrot and noodles in another bowl of iced water; drain. Transfer to a large bowl. Add tomatoes and dressing; toss gently to combine. Sprinkle with shallots.

6 Serve sliced chicken with noodle mixture, mint and lime wedges.

TIPS Chicken supremes are the chicken breast and first wing joint attached with the skin; they are available from gourmet chicken shops and some butchers. You may need to order them. You can brown the chicken in a frying pan, if you prefer.

NUTRITION PER SERVING *32G TOTAL FAT (10.7G SATURATED FAT); 2925KJ (699 CAL); 43.1G CARBOHYDRATE; 54.5G PROTEIN; 10G FIBRE*

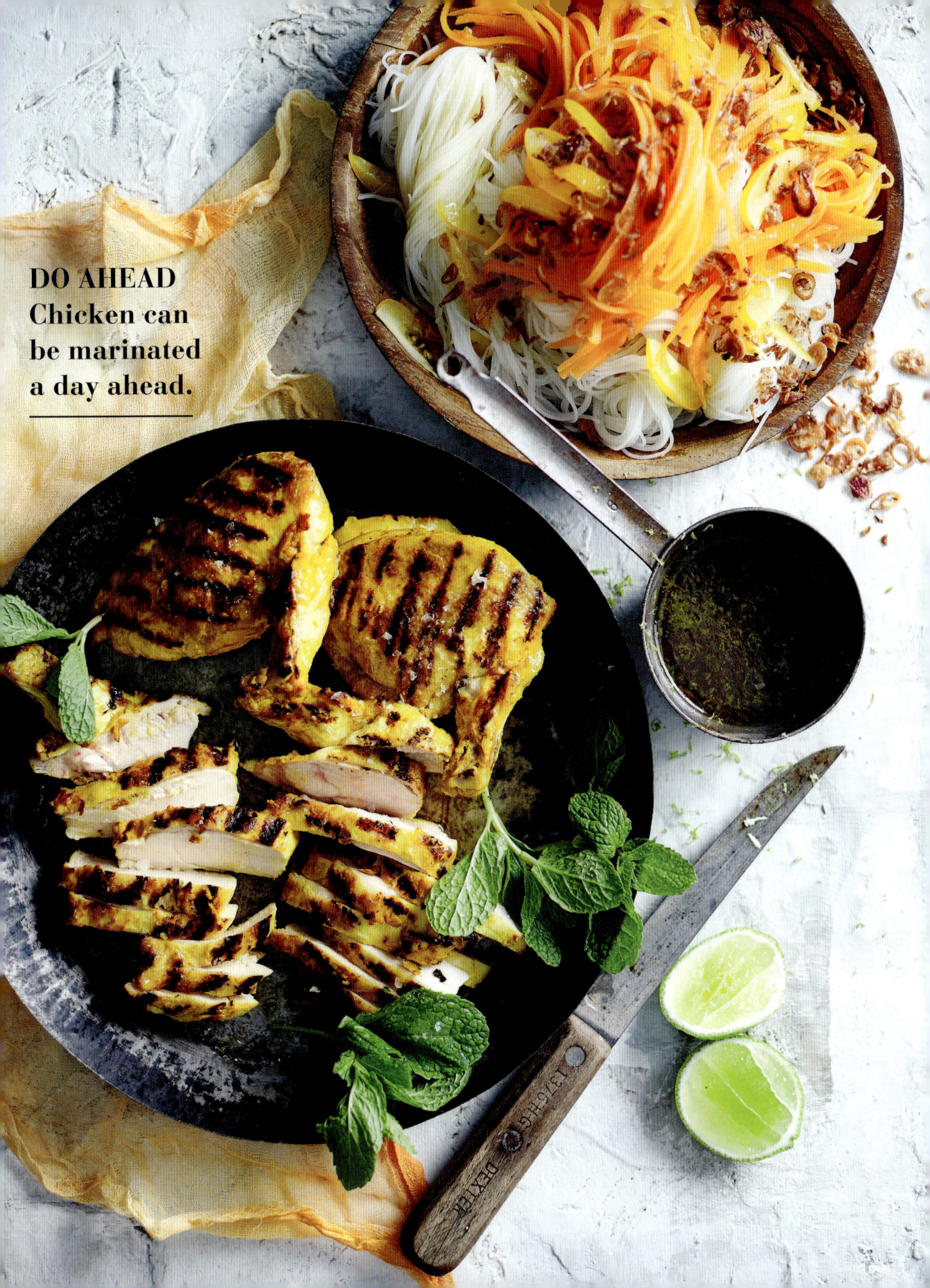

DO AHEAD
Chicken can be marinated a day ahead.

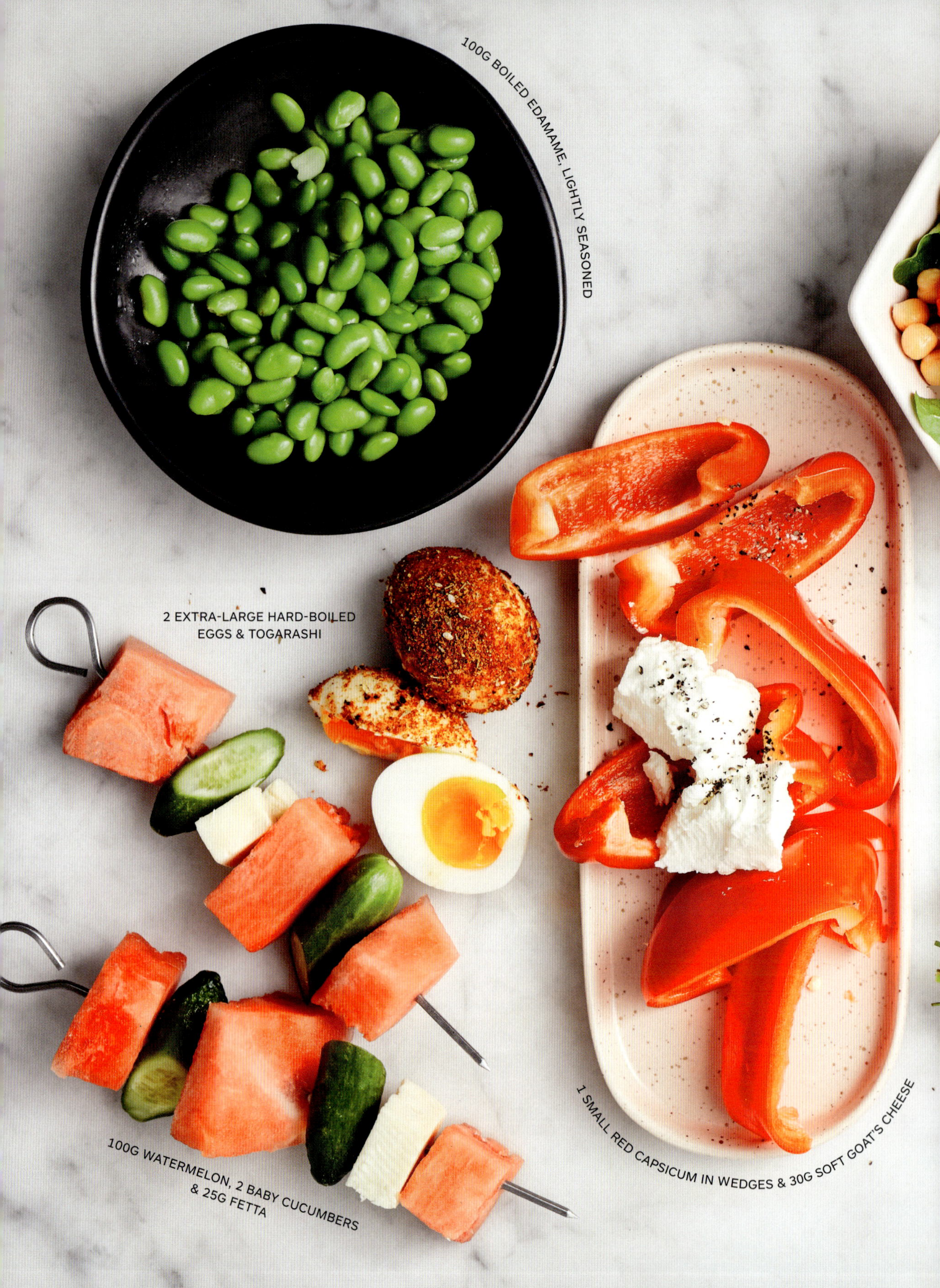
100G BOILED EDAMAME, LIGHTLY SEASONED
2 EXTRA-LARGE HARD-BOILED
EGGS & TOGARASHI
1 SMALL RED CAPSICUM IN WEDGES & 30G SOFT GOAT'S CHEESE
100G WATERMELON, 2 BABY CUCUMBERS
& 25G FETTA

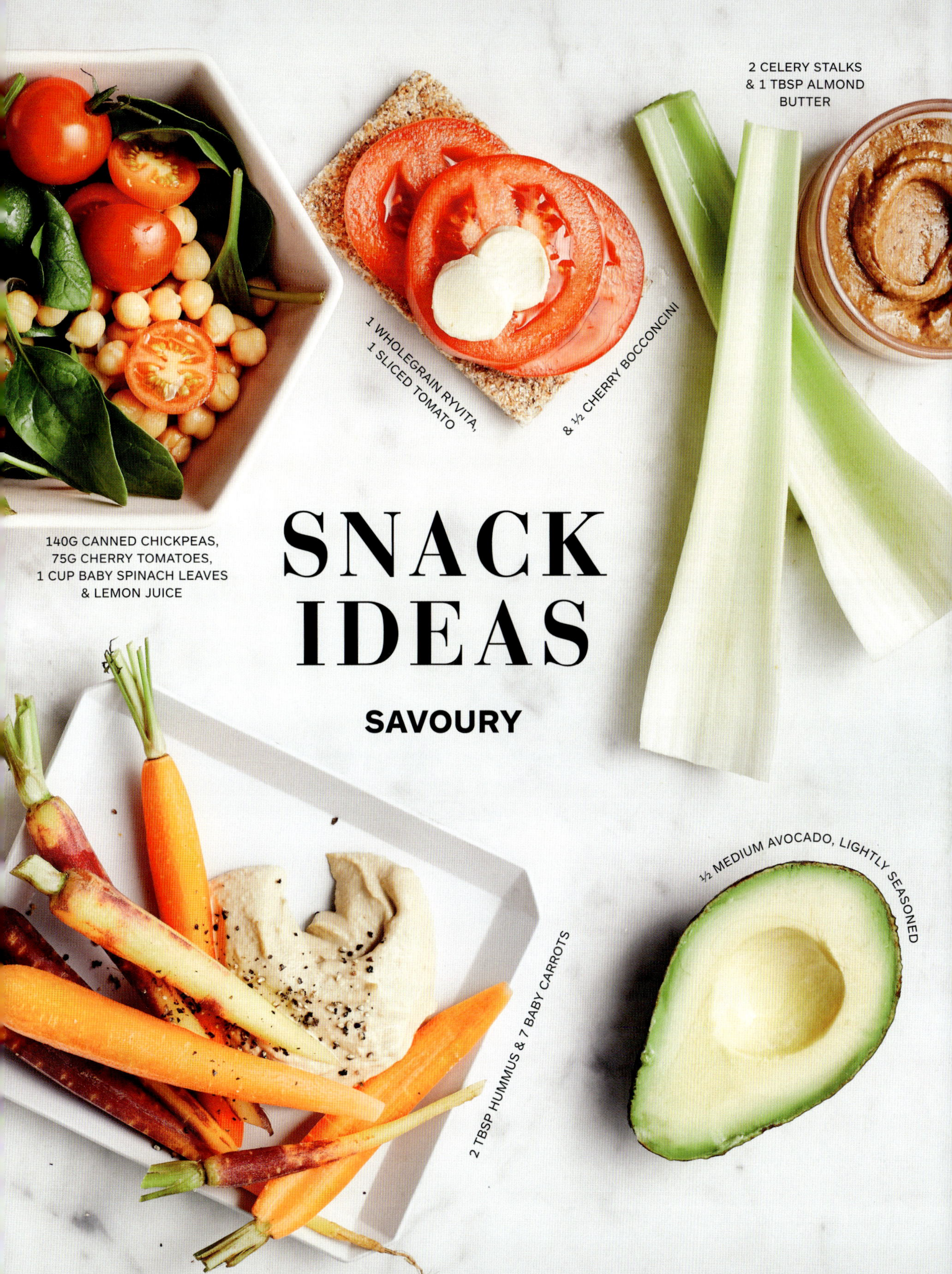
SNACK IDEAS
SAVOURY
140G CANNED CHICKPEAS, 75G CHERRY TOMATOES, 1 CUP BABY SPINACH LEAVES & LEMON JUICE
1 WHOLEGRAIN RYVITA, 1 SLICED TOMATO & ½ CHERRY BOCCONCINI
2 CELERY STALKS & 1 TBSP ALMOND BUTTER
2 TBSP HUMMUS & 7 BABY CARROTS
½ MEDIUM AVOCADO, LIGHTLY SEASONED

LEMONY SPICED CHICKEN WITH BULGUR & BROCCOLINI

PREP + COOK TIME *30 MINUTES (+ REFRIGERATION)*
SERVES *4*

- **2 chicken breast fillets (400g)**
- **4 small cloves garlic**
- **1 tbsp finely grated lemon rind**
- **¼ cup (60ml) lemon juice**
- **1 tsp ground cumin**
- **½ cup (125ml) extra virgin olive oil**
- **1 bunch broccolini (175g), halved lengthways**
- **4 flat mushrooms (320g), cut into thick slices**
- **1 cup (160g) coarse bulgur wheat**
- **120g baby rocket leaves**
- **⅓ cup (50g) pomegranate seeds (arils)**
- **100g store-brought labne**

1 Cut chicken fillets in half horizontally; place in a bowl. Thinly slice 3 cloves garlic; add to chicken. Combine lemon rind and juice, cumin and oil in a jug. Pour ¼ cup of the dressing over chicken; turn to coat chicken.

2 Crush remaining garlic clove into remaining dressing in jug. Place broccolini and mushrooms in another bowl with 2 tablespoons of the remaining dressing; toss to coat. Refrigerate chicken and vegetables for 20 minutes.

3 Meanwhile, place bulgur in a bowl with enough boiling water to cover. Stand, covered, for 10 minutes or until tender. Drain well. Return to bowl.

4 Heat a grill plate (or grill pan) over high heat; cook chicken for 2 minutes each side or until cooked through. Transfer to a plate; rest for 4 minutes. Cook broccolini and mushrooms on grill plate for 2 minutes each side. Cut grilled chicken into thick slices on the diagonal.

5 Add rocket and pomegranate seeds with remaining dressing to bulgur in bowl; toss gently to combine.

6 Serve bulgur mixture with chicken, broccolini and mushrooms; top with dollops of labne. Season.

NUTRITION PER SERVING *34.6G TOTAL FAT (7G SATURATED FAT); 2459KJ (588 CAL); 30.6G CARBOHYDRATE; 33.5G PROTEIN; 8.4G FIBRE*

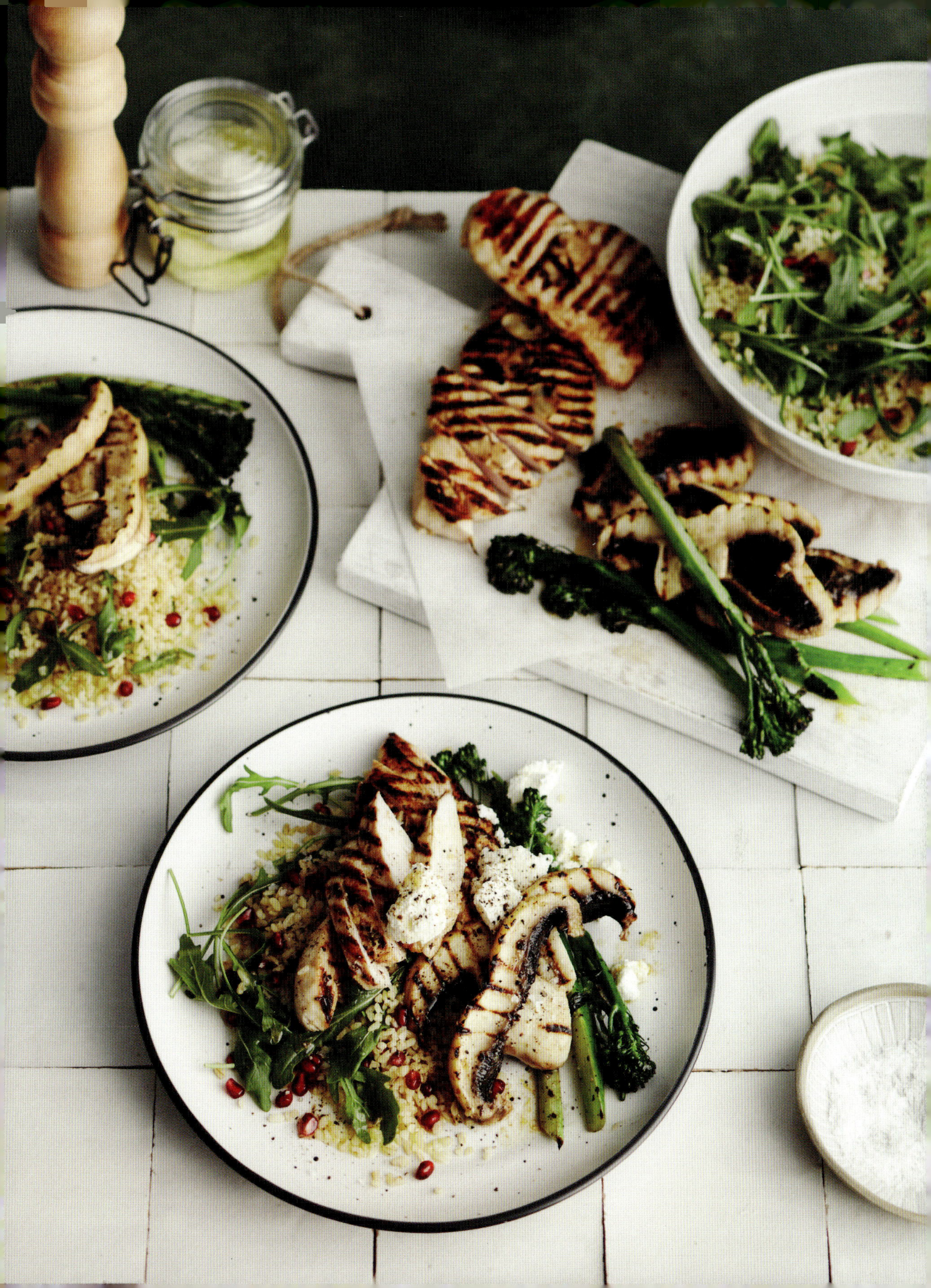

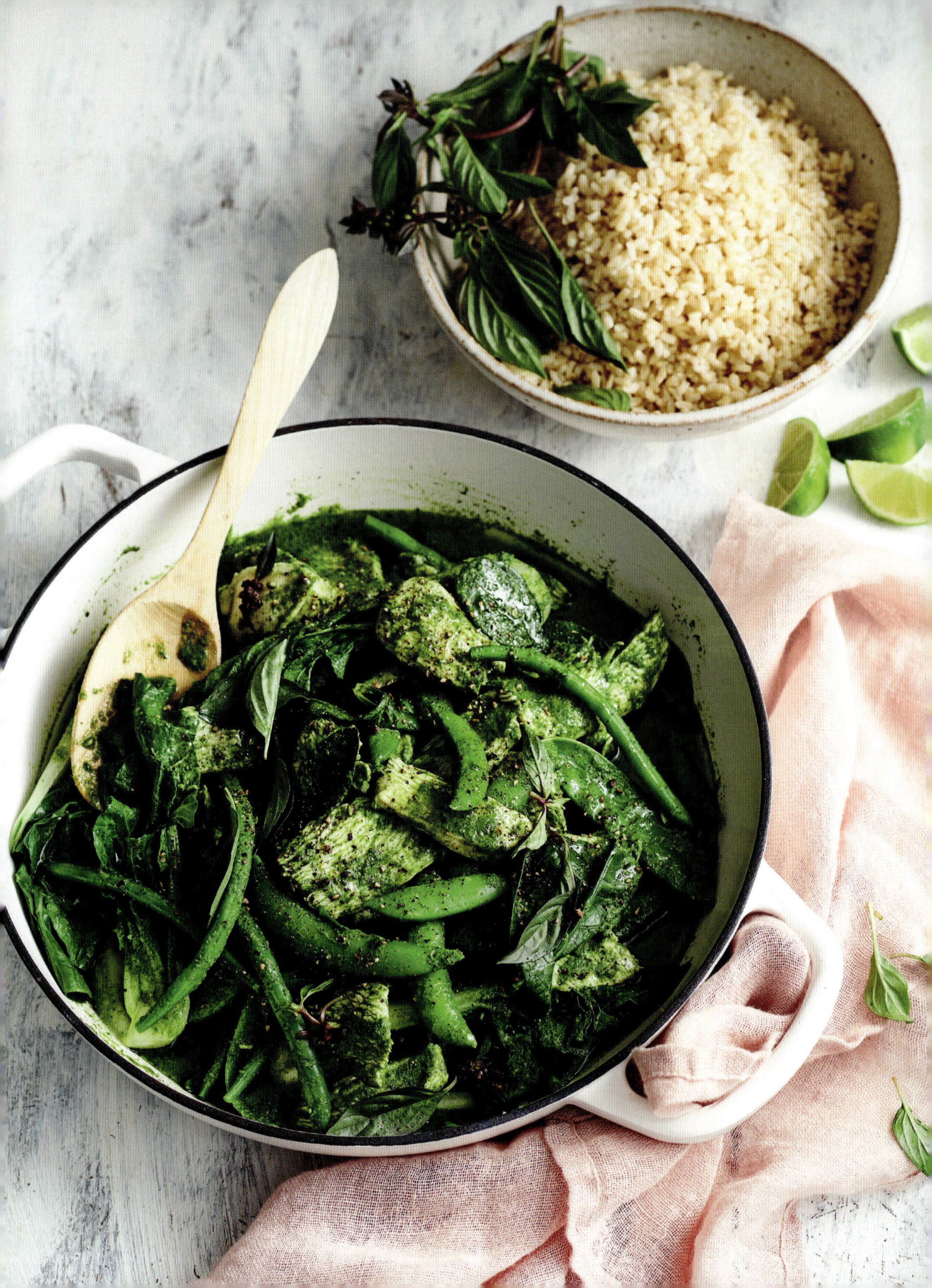

MAKRUT LIME GREEN CHICKEN CURRY

PREP + COOK TIME *45 MINUTES*
SERVES 4

2 cups (400g) doongara low-GI brown rice (see tip)

1 tbsp extra virgin olive oil

⅓ cup (100g) Thai green curry paste

400ml can coconut milk

2 tbsp lime juice

100g baby spinach leaves

3 chicken breast fillets (600g), cut into 5mm thick slices

4 makrut lime leaves

140g baby buk choy, quartered lengthways

150g green beans, trimmed, halved

150g sugar snap peas, trimmed

150g snow peas, trimmed

½ cup Thai basil leaves

lime wedges, to serve

1 Cook rice according to packet directions. Cover to keep warm.

2 Meanwhile, heat oil in a large heavy-based saucepan over medium heat. Add curry paste; cook for 2 minutes or until fragrant. Stir in coconut milk and lime juice. Bring almost to the boil; simmer for 2 minutes. Blend curry mixture and spinach in a blender until as smooth as possible; return to pan.

3 Add chicken and lime leaves to sauce; stir to combine. Bring to the boil. Reduce heat; simmer, covered, for 2 minutes or until chicken is almost cooked. Add buk choy and beans; cook, uncovered, stirring, for 5 minutes or until vegetables are tender. Stir in sugar snap and snow peas; cook for 1 minute or until peas are just tender. Stir in basil.

4 Serve curry with rice and lime wedges.

TIP Doongara rice, grown exclusively in Australia; is a naturally low-GI rice variety available from major supermarkets.

NUTRITION PER SERVING *25G TOTAL FAT (14.2G SATURATED FAT); 1930KJ (461 CAL); 84.6G CARBOHYDRATE; 48.4G PROTEIN; 10.5G FIBRE*

GRILLED CALAMARI WITH CANNELLINI BEAN PUREE

PREP + COOK TIME *55 MINUTES (+ OVERNIGHT SOAKING)*
SERVES *4*

2 cups (400g) dried cannellini beans

2 tbsp extra virgin olive oil

2 medium red onions (340g), chopped

3 cloves garlic, crushed

1 litre (4 cups) vegetable stock

¼ cup (60ml) lemon juice

12 small calamari (1kg)

lemon wedges, to serve

OREGANO SALSA

1 cup firmly packed flat-leaf parsley leaves, chopped finely

½ cup firmly packed oregano leaves, chopped finely

2 green onions, sliced thinly

2 tbsp baby capers

1 long red chilli, seeded, chopped finely

¼ cup (60ml) sherry vinegar

½ cup (125ml) extra virgin olive oil

1 Place cannellini beans in a bowl with enough cold water to cover. Stand to soak overnight. Drain.

2 Heat oil in a saucepan over heat; cook onion and garlic, stirring, for 5 minutes. Add drained beans and stock. Cover pan; bring to the boil. Reduce heat; simmer, covered, for 40 minutes. Drain beans, reserving cooking liquid. Process beans, lemon juice and enough of the reserved cooking liquid until a smooth puree forms. Season; keep warm.

3 Meanwhile, to clean calamari, pull heads and tentacles with the internal sac away from the hood. Cut the tentacles from the head just below the eyes; discard head. Carefully pull out and discard the quill. Remove and discard side fins. Pull skin away from hoods. Wash the hoods and tentacles thoroughly; pat dry with paper towel.

4 Place a cook's knife flat inside one of the calamari hoods. Using a second knife, slice calamari crossways at 1cm intervals (as if you're cutting into rings; the knife will prevent you cutting all the way through the calamari). Repeat with remaining calamari.

5 To make oregano salsa, combine ingredients in a medium bowl; season to taste. (Makes 1 cup.)

6 Heat a grill plate (or grill pan) on high. Place calamari tubes and tentacles into a medium bowl. Add ¼ cup (60ml) of liquid from the salsa; toss to combine. Season. Cook calamari, in batches, for 1 minute on each side or until charred and cooked through.

7 Serve grilled calamari with oregano salsa and bean puree.

NUTRITION PER SERVING *45.8G TOTAL FAT (8.7G SATURATED FAT); 4000KJ (957 CAL); 43.6G CARBOHYDRATE; 67.1G PROTEIN; 33.7G FIBRE*

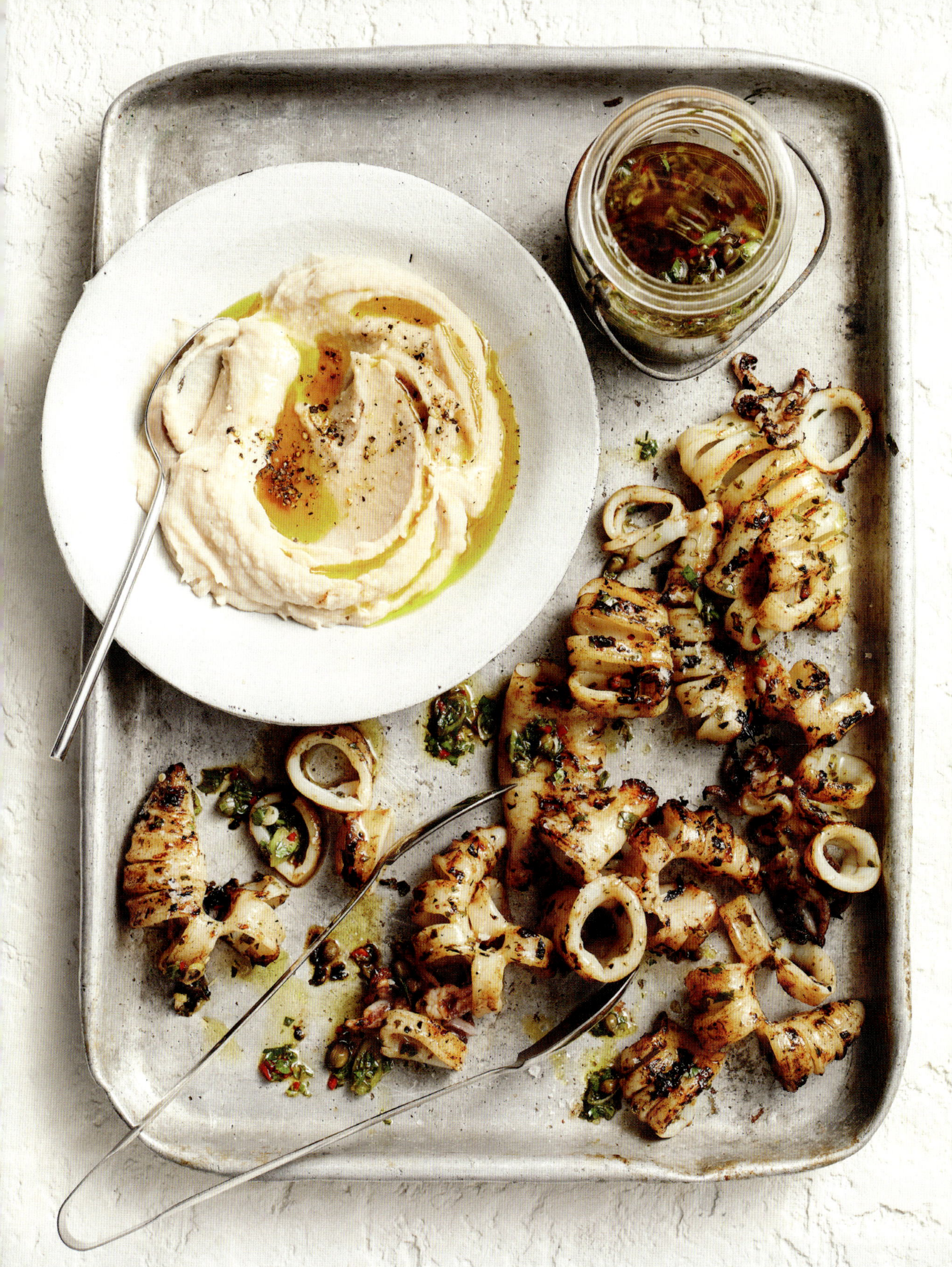

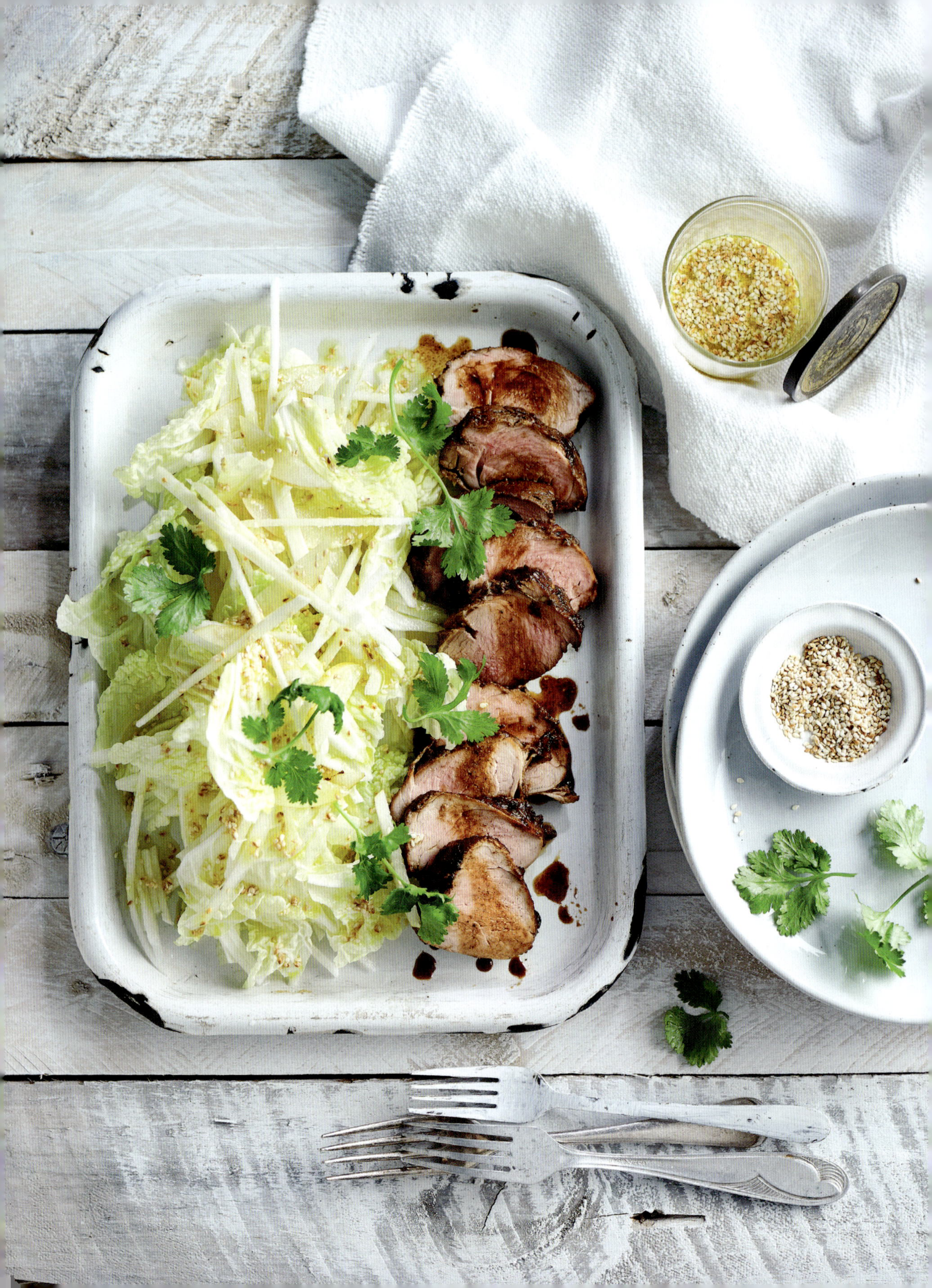

WOMBOK & NASHI SLAW WITH PORK

PREP + COOK TIME *30 MINUTES (+ REFRIGERATION & STANDING)*
SERVES *4*

1 tbsp tamari
1 tbsp sesame oil
1 tsp five-spice powder
1 tsp finely grated lemon rind
600g pork fillet
2 tbsp maple syrup
1 medium jicama (300g), peeled, cut into matchsticks (see tip)
200g wombok, torn
1 medium nashi (200g), sliced thinly
⅓ cup (80ml) lemon juice
½ cup (125ml) extra virgin olive oil
2 tbsp sesame seeds, toasted
¼ cup coriander leaves

1 Preheat oven to 200°C. Line a medium oven tray with baking paper.

2 Combine tamari, sesame oil, five-spice and rind in a large bowl. Trim pork of any fat. Add pork to bowl, turn to coat; season. Cover; refrigerate for 30 minutes.

3 Transfer pork to tray. Roast for 20 minutes or until just cooked through. Transfer pork to a plate; drizzle with half the syrup. Cover loosely with foil; stand for 10 minutes.

4 Meanwhile, combine jicama, wombok and nashi in a bowl. Add combined juice, olive oil, sesame seeds and remaining maple syrup; toss gently to combine. Season.

5 Slice pork; serve with slaw and coriander.

TIP Jicama, pronounced hi-kah-ma, is also known as a yam bean. It's mostly served raw in salads and salsas. Keep it at room temperature or refrigerate once cut. It must be peeled before use.

NUTRITION PER SERVING *38.3G TOTAL FAT (6.1G SATURATED FAT); 2359KJ (564 CAL); 23.4G CARBOHYDRATE; 38.1G PROTEIN; 6.8G FIBRE*

GRILLED FISH & QUINOA SALAD WITH GREEN HUMMUS

PREP + COOK TIME *35 MINUTES*
SERVES *4*

- **⅔ cup (135g) tri-coloured quinoa (see tips)**
- **500g skinless boneless blue-eye trevalla fillets (see tips)**
- **2 tsp olive oil**
- **1 cup flat-leaf parsley leaves, chopped**
- **1 cup coriander leaves, chopped**
- **1 cup mint leaves, chopped**
- **1 tsp ground sumac**
- **2 long green chillies, seeded, chopped finely**
- **½ cup (130g) store-bought hummus**
- **¼ cup (60ml) lemon juice**
- **200g trimmed watercress**
- **200g cherry tomatoes, halved**
- **1 small Lebanese cucumber (100g), halved lengthways, sliced thinly**
- **⅓ cup (50g) pomegranate seeds (arils)**
- **1 tbsp pomegranate molasses**

1 Place quinoa in a sieve and rinse under cold running water. Combine quinoa and 1¼ cups (310ml) water in a medium saucepan over high heat, cover; bring to the boil. Reduce heat to low; cook, covered, for 10 minutes. Stand, covered, for 10 minutes.

2 Meanwhile, preheat a grill plate (or grill pan) on high. Brush fish with oil; cook for 3 minutes each side or until just cooked through. (The cooking time will depend on the thickness of the fish.) Transfer fish to a plate; cover loosely with foil.

3 To make green hummus, process parsley, coriander, mint, sumac, chilli, hummus, 1½ tablespoons water and half the lemon juice until smooth.

4 Place quinoa, watercress, tomatoes, cucumber, pomegranate seeds and remaining lemon juice in a large bowl; toss to combine.

5 Serve fish with quinoa salad; drizzle with green hummus and pomegranate molasses.

TIPS Use red or white quinoa instead of tri-coloured, if preferred. Any firm white fish fillet, such as ling, kingfish or snapper, would work well in this recipe.

NUTRITION PER SERVING *12.1G TOTAL FAT (2.1G SATURATED FAT); 1731KJ (413 CAL); 36.5G CARBOHYDRATE; 34.5G PROTEIN; 9.8G FIBRE*

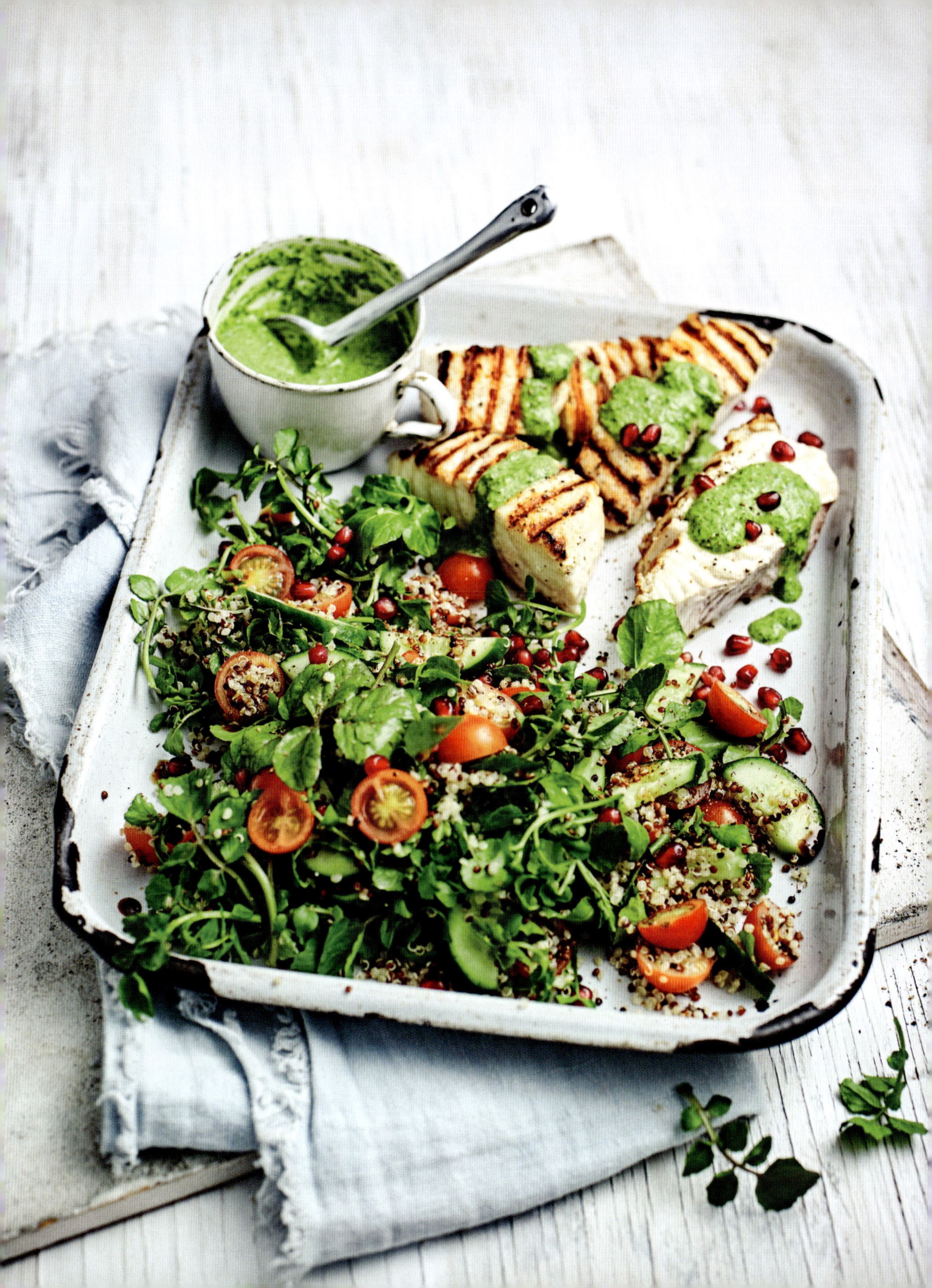

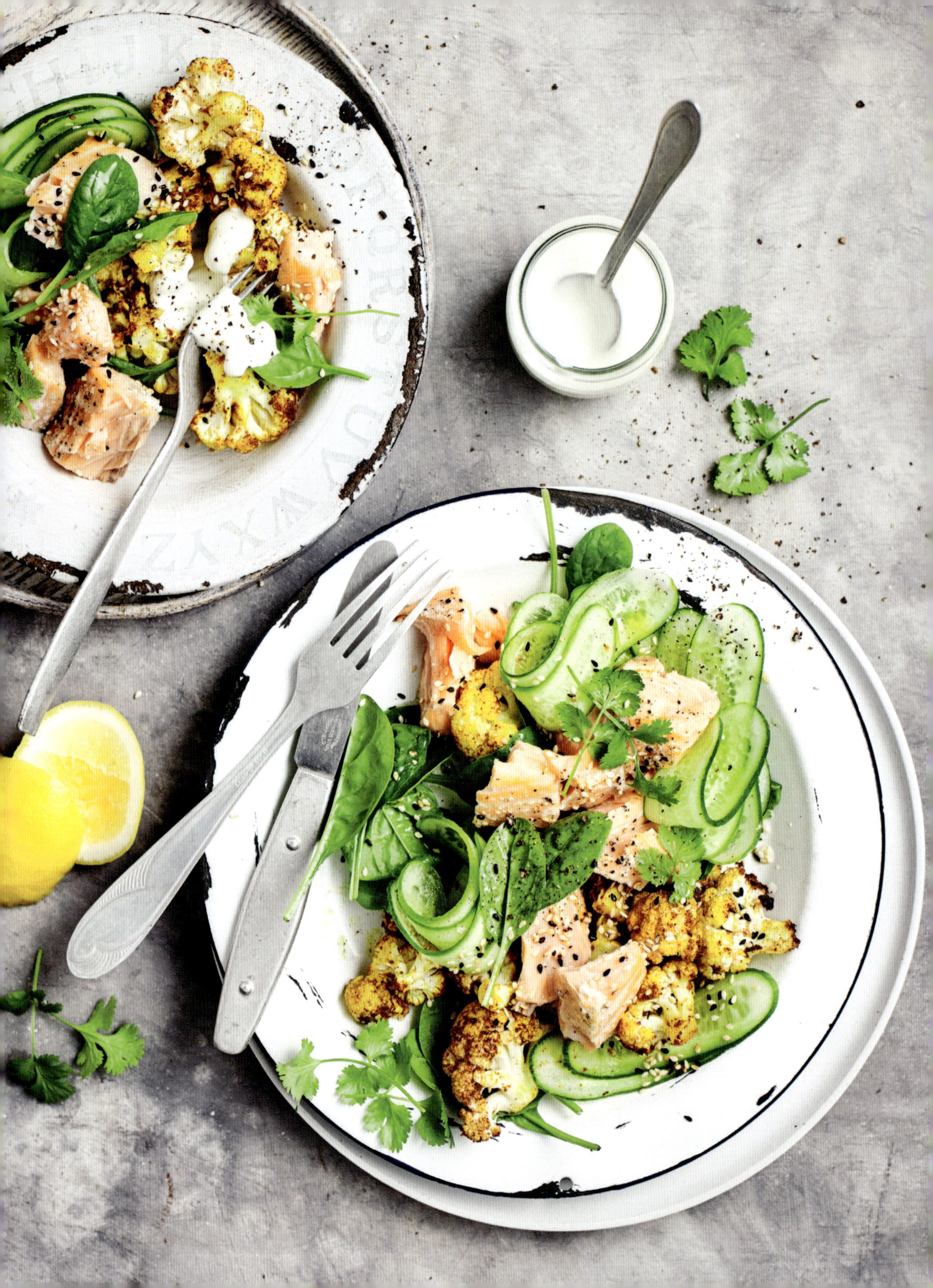

ROAST SALMON WITH SPICED CAULIFLOWER & SPINACH

PREP + COOK TIME *50 MINUTES*
SERVES *4*

- **1.5kg cauliflower, cut into florets**
- **extra virgin olive oil spray**
- **3 tsp garam masala**
- **2 tsp ground turmeric**
- **600g skinless boneless salmon fillets**
- **180g baby spinach leaves**
- **200g baby cucumbers, sliced very thinly lengthways**
- **½ cup coriander leaves**
- **1½ tbsp extra virgin olive oil**
- **2 tbsp lemon juice**
- **½ cup (140g) Greek yoghurt**
- **1 tbsp white sesame seeds, toasted**
- **2 tsp black sesame seeds**
- **1 medium lemon (140g), cut into cheeks**

1 Preheat oven to 200°C. Line two large oven trays with baking paper.

2 Spray cauliflower with oil, combine with garam masala and turmeric in a large bowl; season. Divide cauliflower between trays. Roast for 20 minutes or until starting to brown.

3 Season salmon. Add salmon to trays with cauliflower. Roast for 5 minutes or until cauliflower is golden and salmon is almost cooked through. Transfer cauliflower to a large bowl; cool. Add spinach, cucumber and coriander to cauliflower in bowl. Break salmon into chunks.

4 To make dressing, place olive oil and half the lemon juice in a screw-top jar; shake well. Season to taste. Add dressing to salad; toss to combine.

5 Combine yoghurt and remaining juice in a small bowl; season to taste.

6 Divide salad and salmon among four plates and drizzle with yoghurt mixture; season. Sprinkle with sesame seeds; serve with lemon cheeks.

PREP IT The dressing and yoghurt mixture can be made a day ahead.

NUTRITION PER SERVING *6.4G TOTAL FAT (0.8G SATURATED FAT); 433KJ (103 CAL); 7.7G CARBOHYDRATE; 2.8G PROTEIN; 2.8G FIBRE*

SPICE-RUBBED STEAK WITH SWEET POTATO WEDGES

PREP + COOK TIME *35 MINUTES*
SERVES *4*

800g orange sweet potato, cut into thin wedges

1 tbsp extra virgin olive oil

2 tsp garlic powder

2 tsp smoked paprika

½ tsp cracked black pepper

480g sirloin steaks

extra virgin olive oil spray

1½ tbsp horseradish cream

⅓ cup (95g) low-fat Greek yoghurt

2 cups (50g) trimmed watercress sprigs

1 medium lemon (140g), cut into wedges

2 tbsp finely chopped flat-leaf parsley

1 Preheat oven to 220°C. Line a large oven tray with baking paper.

2 Combine sweet potato wedges and oil in a large bowl. Place on lined tray; season with pepper. Bake for 25 minutes or until golden brown and crisp.

3 Meanwhile, combine garlic powder, paprika and pepper in a small bowl. Rub over both sides of the steaks. Heat a chargrill pan over medium-high heat. Spray lightly with oil spray. Cook steaks for 3 minutes each side for medium-rare or until cooked to your liking. Transfer to a plate to rest.

4 Combine horseradish cream and yoghurt in a small bowl.

5 Serve steaks with sweet potato wedges, horseradish yoghurt, watercress sprigs and lemon wedges. Sprinkle with parsley.

NUTRITION PER SERVING *10.3G TOTAL FAT (2.6G SATURATED FAT); 1488KJ (355 CAL); 32.1G CARBOHYDRATE; 28.2G PROTEIN; 8.1G FIBRE*

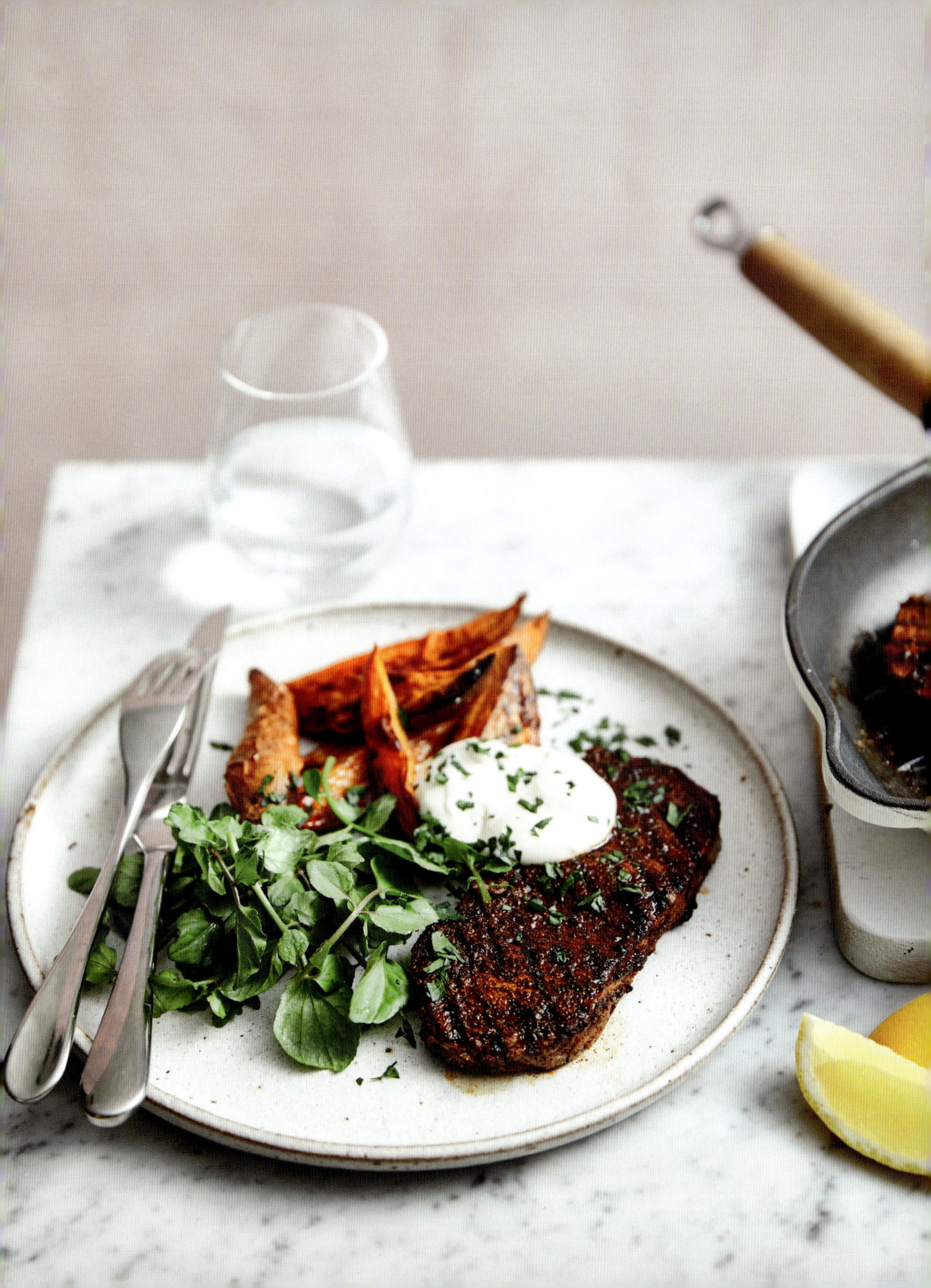

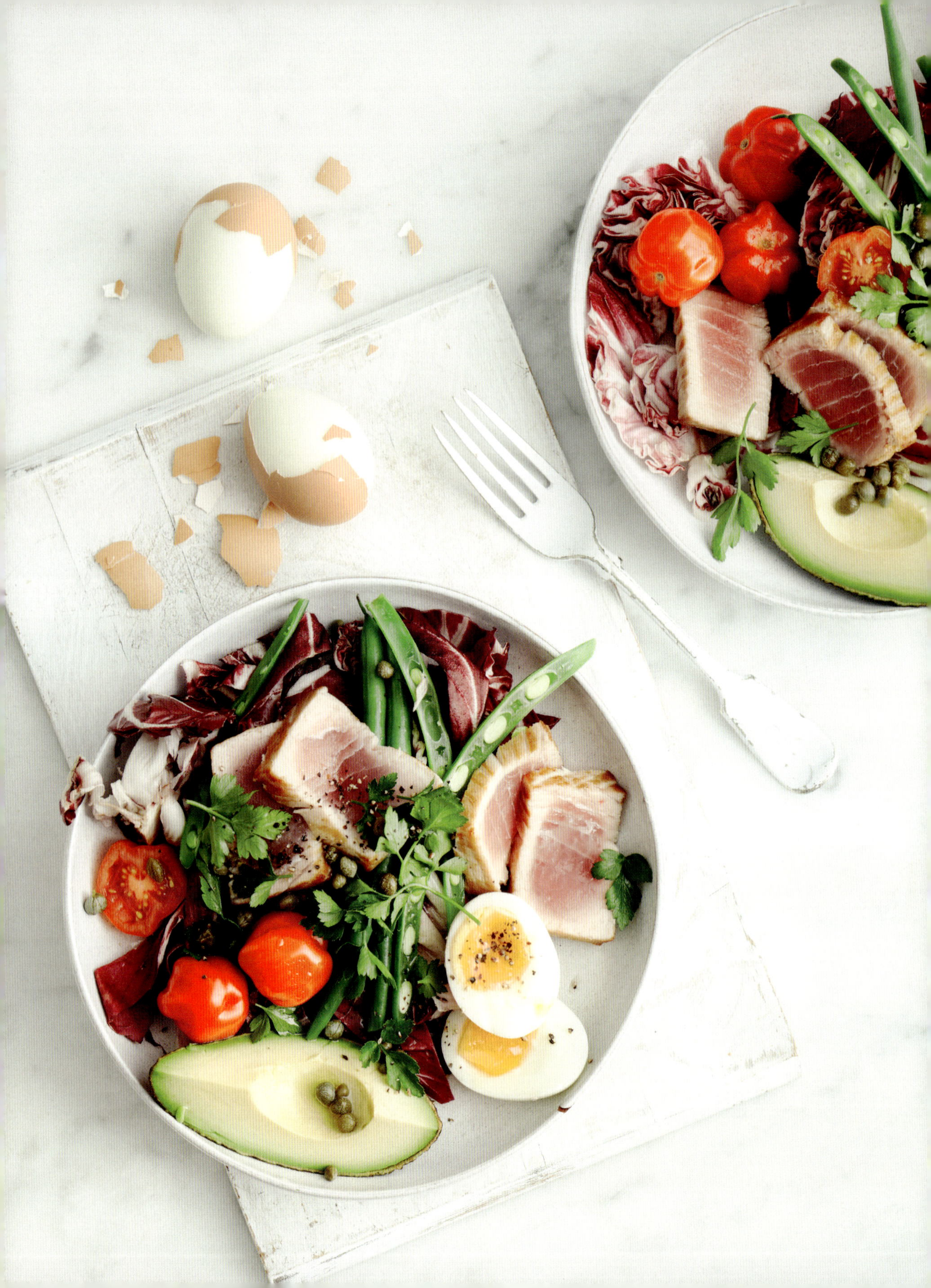

NIÇOISE SALAD

PREP + COOK TIME *30 MINUTES*
SERVES *4*

- **4 extra-large eggs (60g each)**
- **200g green beans, trimmed, halved lengthways**
- **¼ cup (60ml) extra virgin olive oil**
- **600g tuna steak**
- **1 tbsp lemon juice**
- **2 tbsp white wine vinegar**
- **1 medium radicchio (200g), sliced thickly**
- **400g baby heirloom tomatoes, halved or left whole**
- **1 medium avocado (250g), quartered**
- **2 tbsp baby capers**
- **¼ cup flat-leaf parsley leaves**

1 Place eggs in a small saucepan, cover with cold water; bring to the boil. Cook for 4 minutes or until medium boiled; drain. Cool eggs in cold water. When cool enough to handle, peel eggs; cut in half.

2 Meanwhile, boil, steam or microwave beans until just tender; drain. Rinse under cold water; drain.

3 Rub 1 tablespoon of the oil all over tuna; season. Cook tuna on a heated oiled grill plate (or grill pan) over high heat, for 1 minute each side or until seared. Remove from heat; rest, covered, for 5 minutes before slicing.

4 To make dressing, whisk remaining oil with lemon juice and vinegar in a small bowl.

5 Divide radicchio, beans, tomatoes, avocado and eggs among bowls. Top with tuna, capers and parsley; drizzle with dressing. Season.

VARIATION For a salmon Niçoise: rub 4 x 150g pin-boned salmon fillets with oil; cook, skin-side down, in a frying pan over medium heat for 4 minutes or until skin is crisp and browned. Turn, cook for 1 minute or until cooked as desired.

TIP Substitute fresh tuna with drained tuna in springwater for a faster option.

NUTRITION PER SERVING *28.8G TOTAL FAT (5.1G SATURATED FAT); 2018KJ (482 CAL); 5G CARBOHYDRATE; 46G PROTEIN; 9.7G FIBRE*

OCEAN TROUT WITH PISTACHIO & OLIVE TAPENADE

PREP + COOK TIME *30 MINUTES*
SERVES *4*

1 medium lemon (140g)

1 cup (180g) pitted green Sicilian olives

45g pistachio dukkah

1 cup flat-leaf parsley leaves, plus ⅓ cup extra to serve

¼ cup (60ml) extra virgin olive oil

4 x 200g ocean trout fillets

⅔ cup (60g) rolled oats

300g green beans, trimmed

150g sugar snap peas

½ bunch silverbeet (375g), cut in 4cm pieces

1 tbsp poppy seeds

1 Preheat oven to 200°C. Line an oven tray with baking paper.

2 Remove rind from the lemon using a zesting tool (alternatively, finely grate the rind). Juice lemon; you need 1 tablespoon of juice.

3 Process olives, dukkah, parsley, the lemon juice, 1 tablespoon of the oil and 1 tablespoon of water until it forms a fine paste.

4 Place trout fillets, skin-side down, on lined tray. Combine ⅓ cup of olive tapenade with the oats; press mixture evenly on the fillets. Bake for 12 minutes or until almost cooked through. Rest, loosely covered, for 5 minutes.

5 Meanwhile, cook beans, peas and silverbeet together in a large saucepan of boiling salted water for 1 minute; drain well. Place vegetables in a large bowl with lemon rind, poppy seeds and remaining oil, season; toss to combine.

6 Serve trout and vegetables topped with extra parsley leaves and remaining tapenade.

NUTRITION PER SERVING *43.6G TOTAL FAT (10.7G SATURATED FAT); 2926KJ (699 CAL); 19.5G CARBOHYDRATE; 50.2G PROTEIN; 17.6G FIBRE*

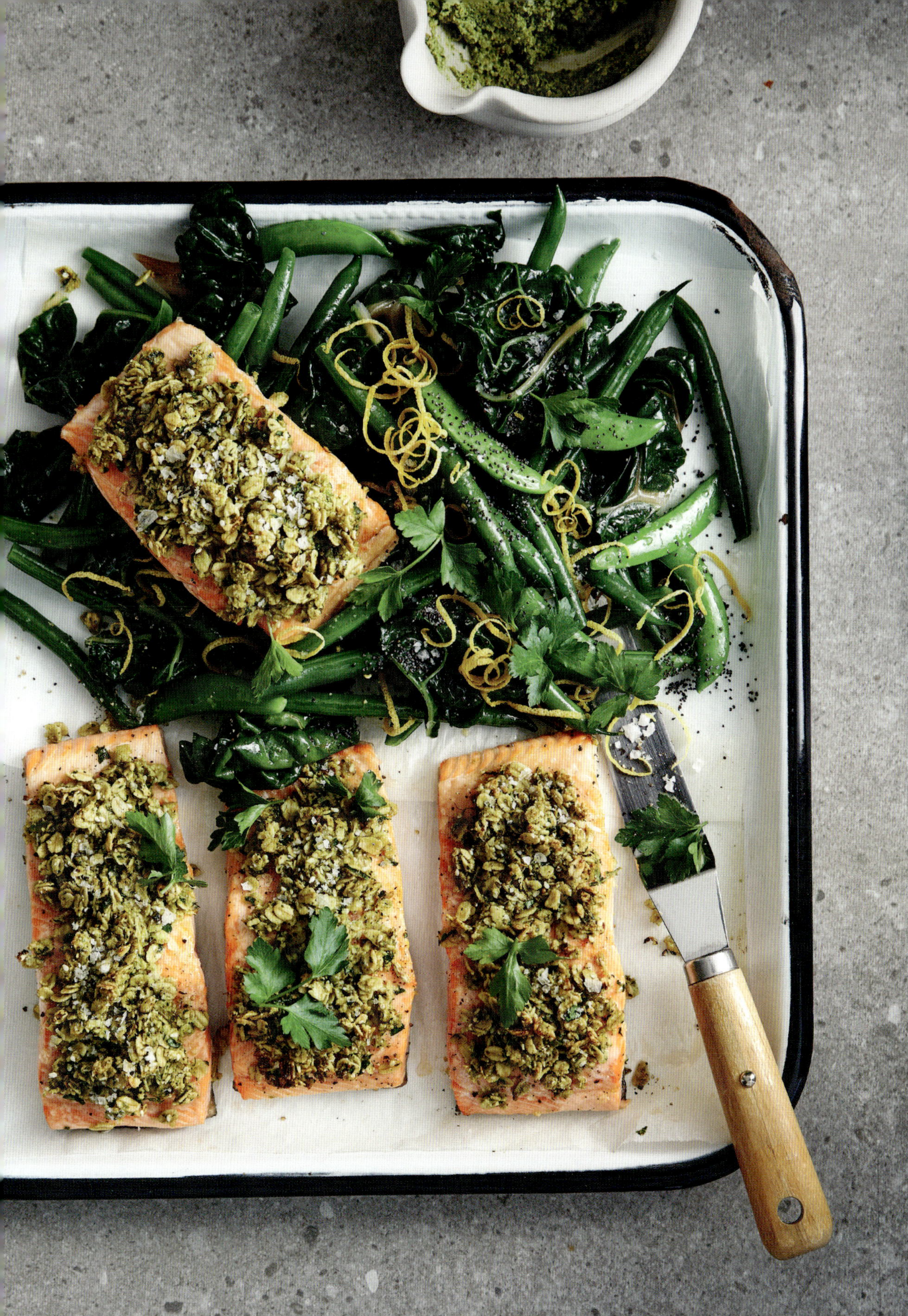

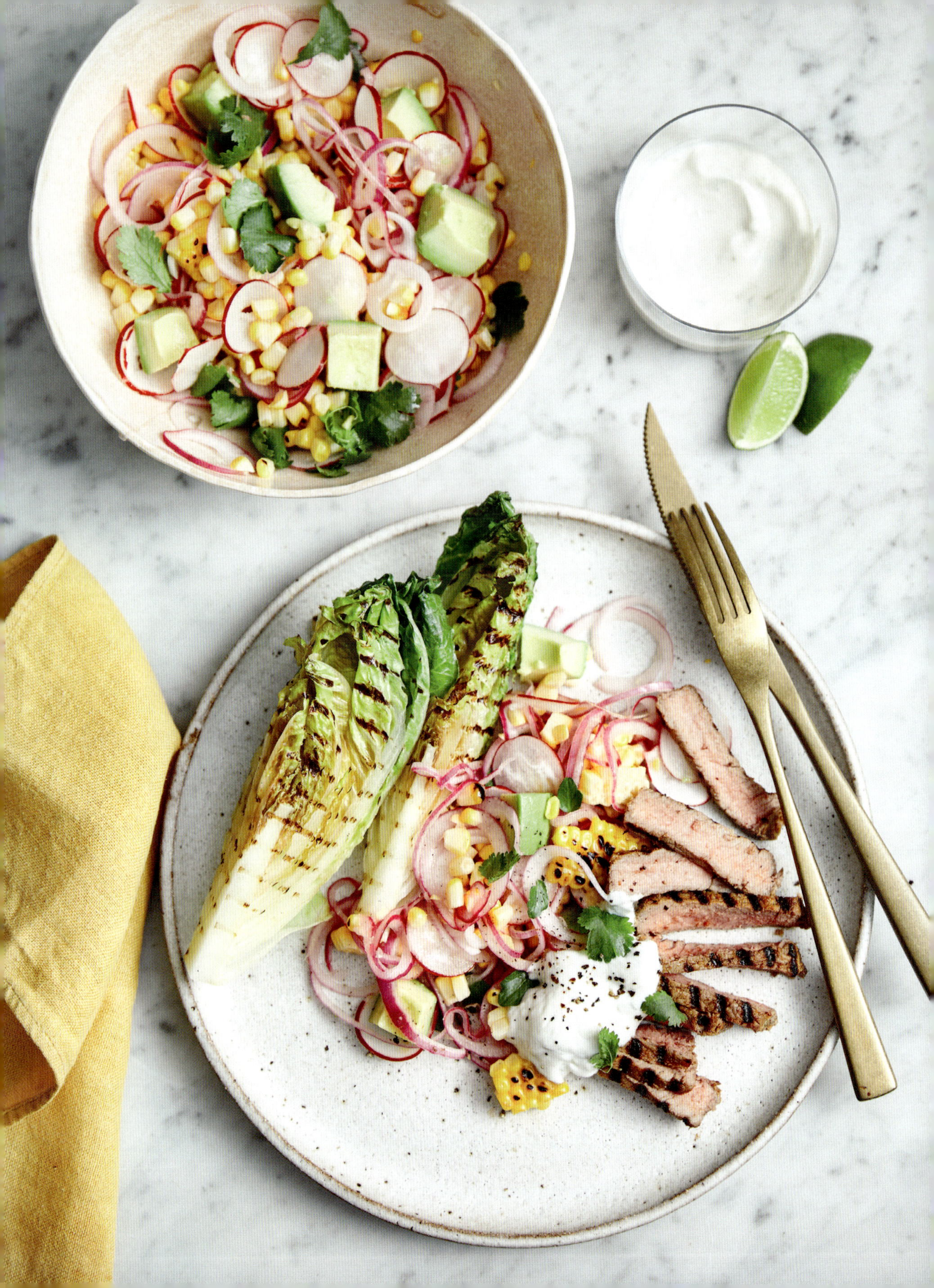

MEXICAN-STYLE STEAK WITH GRILLED CORN SALAD

PREP + COOK TIME *40 MINUTES (+ STANDING)*
SERVES 4

- 1 tbsp extra virgin olive oil
- 3 cloves garlic, crushed
- 2 limes (130g), rind grated finely, juiced (see tips)
- 1 tsp smoked paprika
- ½ tsp ground cumin
- 550g sirloin steak
- extra virgin olive oil spray
- 2 trimmed corn cobs (500g)
- 1 small red onion (100g), sliced very thinly
- 2 baby cos lettuce (300g), quartered lengthways
- ⅓ cup (95g) high-protein natural yoghurt
- 1 medium avocado (250g), cut into 2cm pieces
- 4 small radishes (60g), sliced thinly
- 1 cup coriander leaves

1 Preheat a grill plate (or grill pan) to high. Combine half the oil, 2 of the crushed garlic cloves, half the lime rind and juice, and the spices in a shallow bowl. Add steak, season with pepper; turn to coat. Stand for 15 minutes.

2 Spray corn cobs lightly with oil spray; cook in chargrill pan, turning occasionally, for 8 minutes or until charred. When cool enough to handle, cut the kernels from cob and place in a medium bowl.

3 Meanwhile, combine onion and remaining lime juice in a small bowl. Stand for 10 minutes to lightly pickle.

4 Spray cos lettuce quarters with oil spray; cook, cut-side down in grill pan, for 2 minutes or until lightly charred.

5 Drizzle the steak with remaining oil. Cook steak in grill pan for 4 minutes each side for medium-rare. Transfer to a plate. Rest for 5 minutes; thinly slice.

6 Meanwhile, drain onion, reserving liquid. Squeeze onion dry and add to corn in bowl. Combine yoghurt, reserved pickling liquid and remaining garlic and lime rind in a small bowl; season to taste.

7 Add avocado, radish and coriander to corn mixture; toss to combine. Season. Divide cos lettuce, steak and corn salad among plates; drizzle with yoghurt mixture to serve.

TIPS You will need about 2 tablespoons of lime juice in this recipe. If you have one, use a mandoline to thinly slice onion and radish.

NUTRITION PER SERVING *20.2G TOTAL FAT (4.5G SATURATED FAT); 1653KJ (395 CAL); 15G CARBOHYDRATE; 33.2G PROTEIN; 9.5G FIBRE*

GREEK LAMB SALAD

PREP + COOK TIME *40 MINUTES (+ REFRIGERATION)*
SERVES *4*

- **3 large potatoes (900g), unpeeled, cut into 1cm slices**
- **3 cloves garlic, crushed**
- **3 tsp oregano leaves**
- **½ cup (125ml) extra virgin olive oil**
- **2 x 300g pieces lamb backstraps**
- **250g cherry truss tomatoes**
- **½ cup (80g) pitted Kalamata olives, halved**
- **125g fetta, crumbled**
- **¼ cup (60ml) balsamic glaze**
- **120g mixed baby spinach and rocket leaves**

1 Boil, steam or microwave potato until tender; drain. Cool slightly.

2 Meanwhile, combine garlic, 2 teaspoons chopped oregano and 2 tablespoons of the oil in a large bowl; season. Add lamb; turn to coat. Cover; refrigerate for 30 minutes.

3 Cook lamb in a heated non-stick frying pan over high heat for 4 minutes each side or until cooked as desired. Transfer to a plate; cover to keep warm. Wipe pan clean.

4 Heat 2 tablespoons of the oil in cleaned pan over high heat; cook potato slices, in batches, for 2 minutes each side or until golden. Transfer to a plate; season. Cover to keep warm.

5 Brush tomatoes with 1 tablespoon of the oil; cook in same pan for 2 minutes or until starting to soften. Season.

6 Arrange sliced lamb, potato and tomatoes on a large platter. Top with olives, fetta and remaining oregano. Drizzle with combined balsamic glaze and remaining oil; season. Serve with salad leaves.

NUTRITION PER SERVING *49.5G TOTAL FAT (12.8G SATURATED FAT); 3451KJ (825 CAL); 40.8G CARBOHYDRATE; 55.8G PROTEIN; 7G FIBRE*

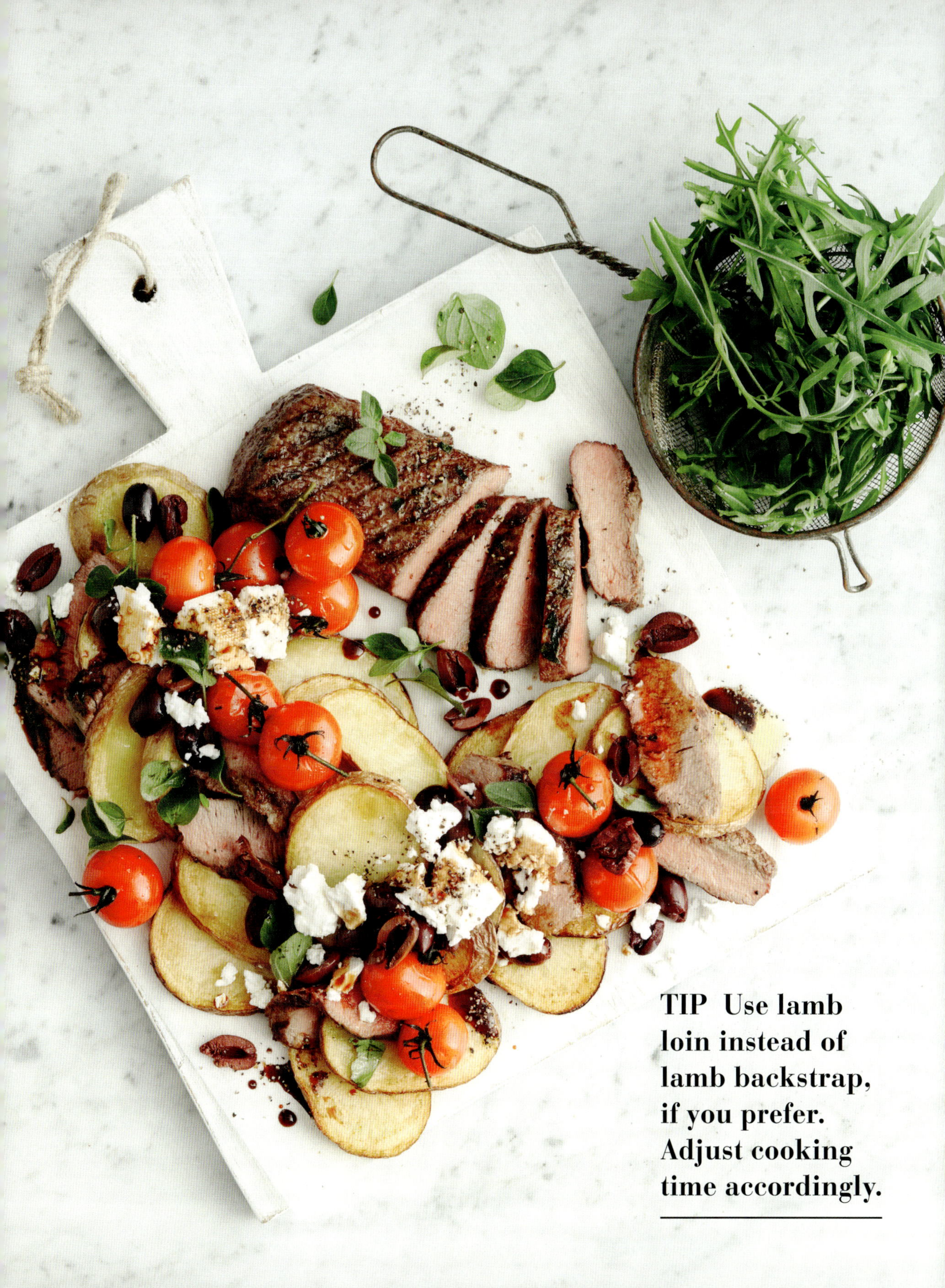

TIP Use lamb loin instead of lamb backstrap, if you prefer. Adjust cooking time accordingly.

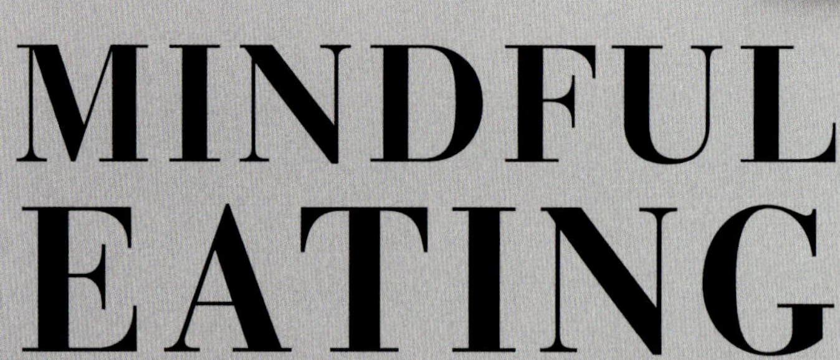

MINDFUL EATING

Let's face it. We've been told 100 times or more what to eat for good health. We know we need to eat more vegetables, cut back on refined sugar, and maybe drink a little less. So what's stopping us? Our mindfulness.

When it comes to losing weight, it's definitely not simply due to a lack of knowledge or willpower. It often comes down to our attention to food. How often do you pay attention to what you're eating? The food and drink you decide to put in your body? What motivates you to eat certain foods?

WHAT IS MINDFUL EATING?

Mindfulness means focusing on the present moment, while calmly accepting your feelings, thoughts and bodily sensations. It also encompasses how the food you eat affects the world, i.e. sustainability and ethical considerations.

The focus of mindful eating isn't deprivation. Mindfulness allows you to indulge without guilt, and to free yourself from the 'diet' mentality. You can get healthy, lose weight, maintain your weight loss and still have a social life... when you start eating with purpose.

By allowing yourself to be aware of what you're eating and why you choose to eat it, you can change your relationship with your food. What did you choose to eat and why? Is it because of true hunger? Or boredom, stress, resentment, sadness, or loneliness? Are you being kind or punishing yourself?

Nurturing your body with a balanced diet rich in colour, variety and plant foods will always be the foundation for healthy eating, but by practising mindful eating around your favourite treat foods, you learn to enjoy them for what they are, appreciate and enjoy the indulgence, and reduce the chances of mindlessly overdoing it.

Follow these six tips to help you start eating more mindfully:

1. SHOP WITH A LIST.

Plan out your meals and snacks as much as you can each week. Prioritise fresh produce and wholesome pantry staples, then stick to your list. It helps to minimise impulse buying, and avoids last-minute decision making at meal times when you're hungry!

2. EAT REGULARLY.

Try and have healthy snacks at the ready to prevent ravenous hunger. Eating too quickly and making poor food choices because you're so hungry is not great for your digestion or your waistline.

3. EMBRACE YOUR INNER FOOD CRITIC.

Take the time to pay attention to the colours, textures, and aromas the different foods have, and savour the flavours as you chew.

4. SAY THANK YOU.

Right before you eat, say a little thank you (you can do it silently) as you contemplate who and what went into bringing the meal together, and appreciate the opportunity to enjoy it and the people you're sharing it with.

5. SLOW DOWN.

Cut your food into smaller pieces and chew thoroughly with each mouthful. Sit when eating and make time to make it an occasion where you pay attention, away from your phone and tv screen. You'll taste more and it will help with digestion too.

6. USE SMALLER UTENSILS.

Opt for entree-sized plates, small dessert bowls and smaller forks and spoons to help you go slow and trick your mind into thinking you're eating more.

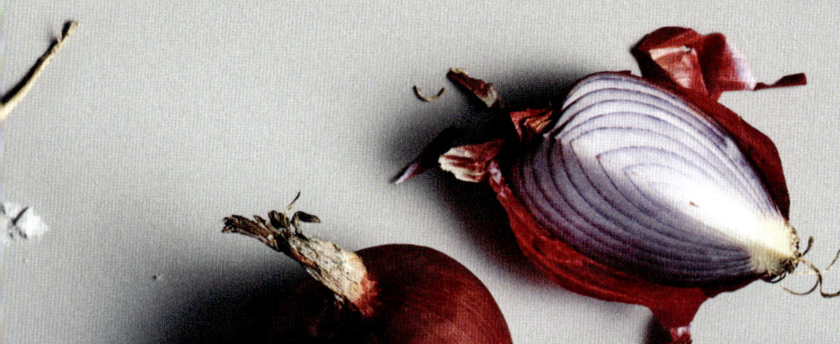

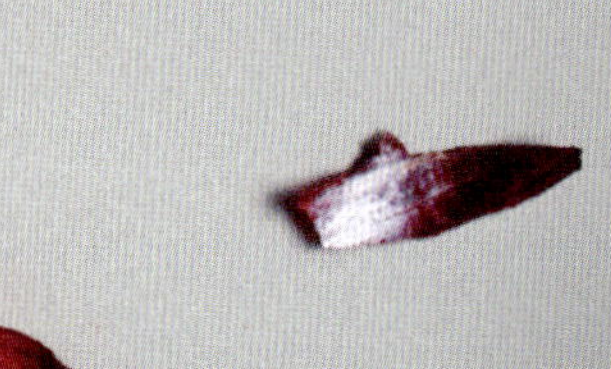

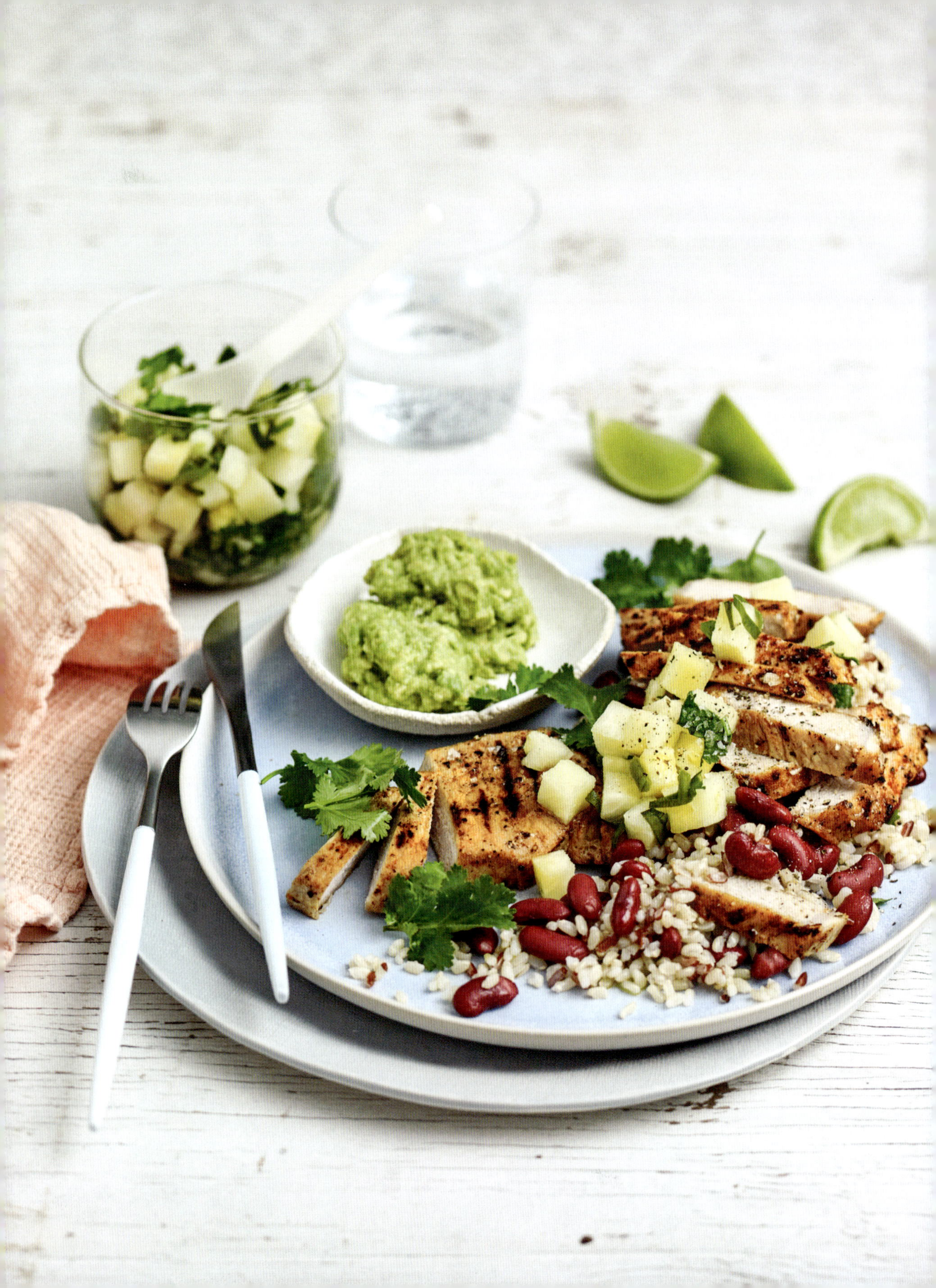

MEXICAN PORK SALAD WITH PINEAPPLE SALSA

PREP + COOK TIME *45 MINUTES*
SERVES *4*

1½ cups (300g) brown rice

500g pork loin steaks

1 tbsp Mexican spice mix

2 tbsp extra virgin olive oil

2 large avocados (640g)

2 tbsp lime juice

400g can red kidney beans, drained, rinsed

coriander leaves and lime wedges, to serve

PINEAPPLE SALSA

1 small pineapple (900g), peeled, cored, diced (see tip)

2 green onions, chopped finely

1 fresh jalapeño chilli, seeded, chopped finely

¼ cup (60ml) ginger kombucha

1 tbsp lime juice

¼ cup chopped coriander

1 To make pineapple salsa, combine ingredients in a medium bowl. Cover; refrigerate until required. (Makes 2½ cups.)

2 Place rice and 3 cups (750ml) water in a large saucepan; bring to the boil. Reduce heat to low and cook, covered, for 25 minutes. Remove from the heat; stand for 5 minutes. Fluff rice with a fork; set aside to cool.

3 Sprinkle pork with spice mix; season. Heat oil in a large heavy-based frying pan over high heat; cook pork for 2 minutes each side or until cooked to your liking. Cover loosely with foil; rest for 2 minutes. Slice pork.

4 Mash avocado and lime juice in a medium bowl until smooth. Season to taste.

5 Combine rice and beans in a large bowl; season to taste.

6 Divide pork, rice mixture, avocado mixture and pineapple salsa among plates. Sprinkle with coriander; season Serve with lime wedges.

TIP The trimmed, peeled and cored pineapple yields about 650g diced flesh.

NUTRITION PER SERVING *35.6G TOTAL FAT (5.7G SATURATED FAT); 3594KJ (859 CAL); 76.3G CARBOHYDRATE; 44.4G PROTEIN; 24G FIBRE*

KOREAN FISH BURGERS WITH KIMCHI SLAW

PREP + COOK TIME *25 MINUTES*
SERVES *4*

2 x 300g skinless boneless salmon fillets

2 tsp sesame oil

2 green onions, sliced thinly, green tops reserved (see tips)

¾ cup (210g) high-protein natural yoghurt

½ clove garlic, crushed

2 tbsp gochujang (see tips)

1 tbsp rice wine vinegar

1 cup (100g) kimchi, chopped

1 cup (150g) kale slaw mix

4 wholegrain or wholemeal buns (280g), split horizontally

4 baby cucumbers (120g), cut lengthways into quarters

lemon wedges, to serve

1 Preheat oven grill to high. Line an oven tray with foil.

2 Cut fish fillets in half crossways; place on lined tray. Brush fish with sesame oil and top with the sliced green onion; season. Place under grill for 8 minutes or until fish is cooked through.

3 Meanwhile, combine yoghurt, garlic, gochujang and vinegar in a small bowl. Combine kimchi and kale slaw mix in a medium bowl.

4 Place bun halves, cut-side up, on an oven tray; place under grill until toasted.

5 Divide kimchi slaw mixture among bun bases; drizzle with yoghurt mixture.
Top with fish, reserved green onion tops (see tips) and bun tops.
Serve with cucumber and lemon wedges.

TIPS Cut the reserved green onion tops into 5cm lengths; then shred finely. Place in iced water for 5 minutes to curl; drain.
Gochujang is a Korean red chilli paste, available from Asian supermarkets.

NUTRITION PER SERVING *29.9G TOTAL FAT (6.5G SATURATED FAT); 2598KJ (621 CAL); 38.9G CARBOHYDRATE; 46.3G PROTEIN; 5.3G FIBRE*

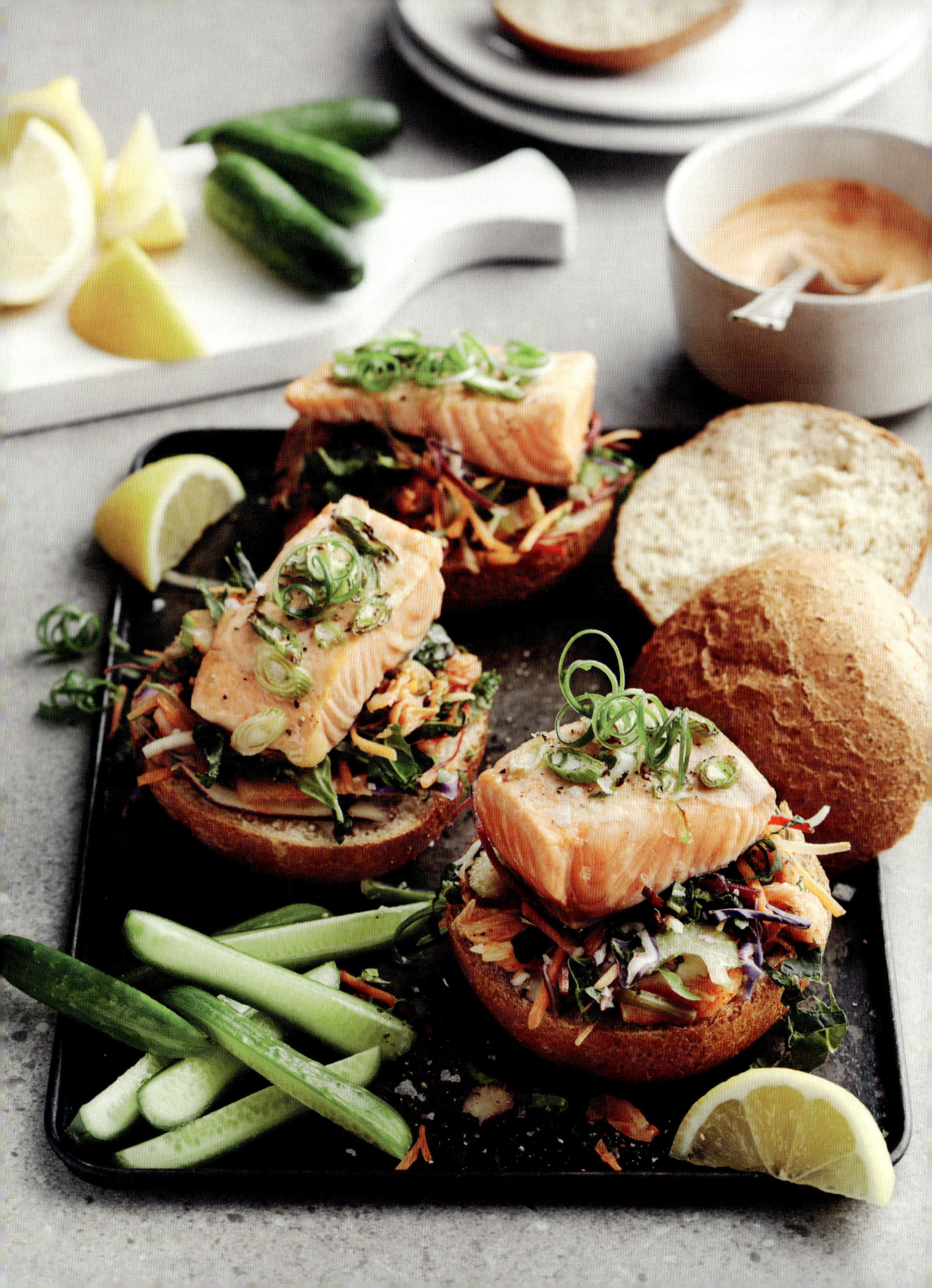

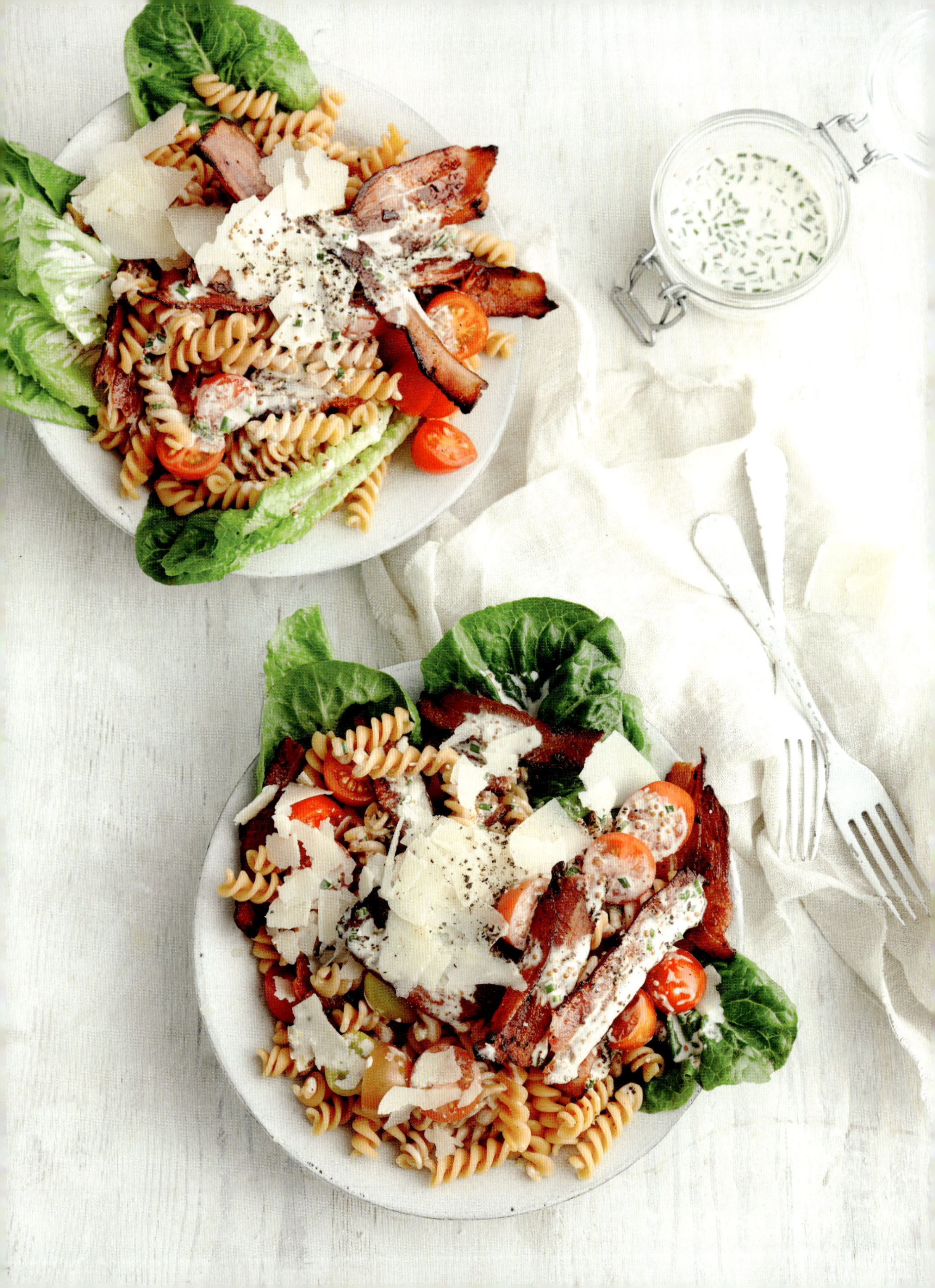

BLT PULSE PASTA SALAD

PREP + COOK TIME *15 MINUTES*
SERVES *4*

250g dried pulse spiral red lentil pasta

250g rindless streaky bacon rashers

1 baby cos lettuce (180g), leaves separated

250g heirloom cherry tomatoes, halved

½ cup (40g) shaved parmesan

DRESSING

¼ cup (75g) whole-egg mayonnaise

2 tsp wholegrain mustard

2 tsp lemon juice

1 tbsp finely chopped chives

1 Cook pasta in a large saucepan of salted boiling water following packet instructions until just tender. Drain; return pasta to pan.

2 Meanwhile, heat a medium non-stick frying pan over high heat; cook bacon for 3 minutes each side or until crisp. Drain on paper towel.

3 To make dressing, whisk ingredients in a bowl until combined. Season to taste.

4 Place pasta and bacon in a large bowl with lettuce and tomatoes; toss gently to combine. Drizzle with half the dressing; top with parmesan. Serve salad with remaining dressing.

TIP We used pulse spiral pasta made from lentils, which is high in fibre, protein and is gluten-free.

NUTRITION PER SERVING *37.8G TOTAL FAT (11.7G SATURATED FAT); 2660KJ (636 CAL); 41.8G CARBOHYDRATE; 29.5G PROTEIN; 5.9G FIBRE*

BAKED FISH 'N' CHIPS

PREP + COOK TIME *40 MINUTES*
SERVES *4*

- 2 large orange sweet potatoes (800g), unpeeled, cut into thin wedges
- 2 tbsp extra virgin olive oil
- 1 tbsp ground cumin
- 1 tbsp ground coriander
- 1 tsp ground turmeric
- 2 tsp coarse cooking salt
- ¼ cup (40g) white sesame seeds
- ⅔ cup (50g) panko (Japanese) breadcrumbs
- ¼ cup (35g) plain flour
- 1 egg
- 800g skinless, boneless firm white fish fillets (see tips)
- lime wedges and dill sprigs, to serve

YOGHURT TARTARE

- ½ cup (140g) Greek yoghurt
- 2 tsp lime juice
- 3 cornichons, chopped finely
- 2 green onions, chopped finely
- 1 tbsp finely chopped dill

1 Preheat oven to 200°C. Line an oven tray with baking paper.

2 Combine sweet potato and half the oil in a medium bowl; season.

3 Place sweet potato, in a single layer, on lined tray; bake for 15 minutes or until browned lightly, cooked through and crisp.

4 Meanwhile, combine spices, salt, seeds and breadcrumbs in a wide shallow bowl. Place flour in another shallow bowl. Lightly beat egg in another shallow bowl. Coat fish in flour, shake off any excess. Dip fish in egg, then in breadcrumb mixture, turning until fish is completely covered.

5 Heat remaining oil in an ovenproof frying pan over medium heat; cook fish for 30 seconds each side or until browned. Transfer frying pan to oven; bake fish for 3 minutes or until just cooked through.

6 Meanwhile, to make yoghurt tartare sauce, combine ingredients in a small bowl; season to taste.

7 Serve fish with chips and yoghurt tartare, sprinkled with extra dill.

TIPS We used flathead fillets here, but you could use snapper, ling, whiting or blue-eye trevalla, if you like. If you don't have an ovenproof frying pan, transfer the fish to an oven tray lined with baking paper before baking. Serve with extra baby gherkins or cornichons and rocket, if you like.

NUTRITION PER SERVING *24G TOTAL FAT (4.7G SATURATED FAT); 2738KJ (654 CAL); 51.9G CARBOHYDRATE; 53.3G PROTEIN; 8.4G FIBRE*

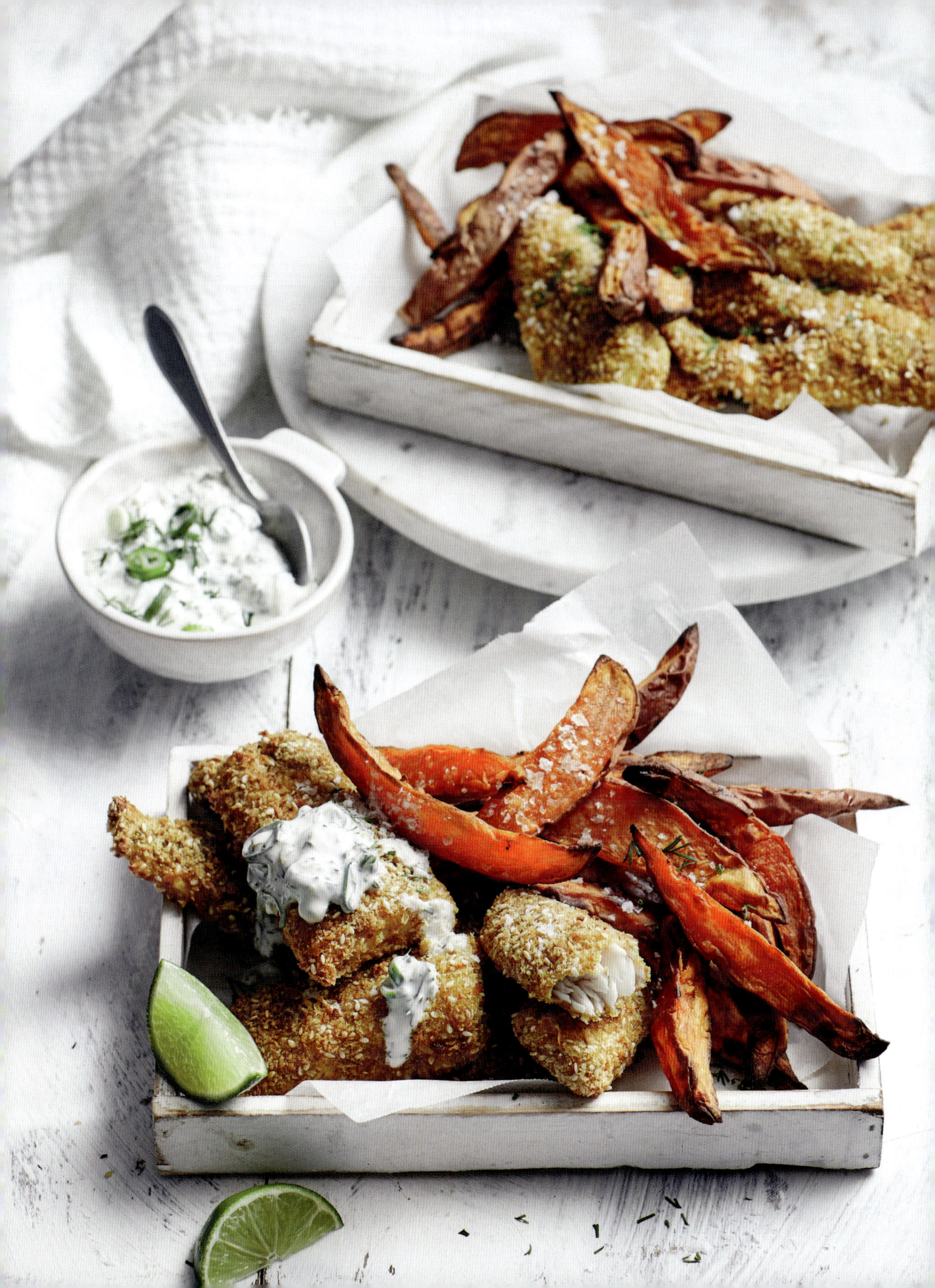

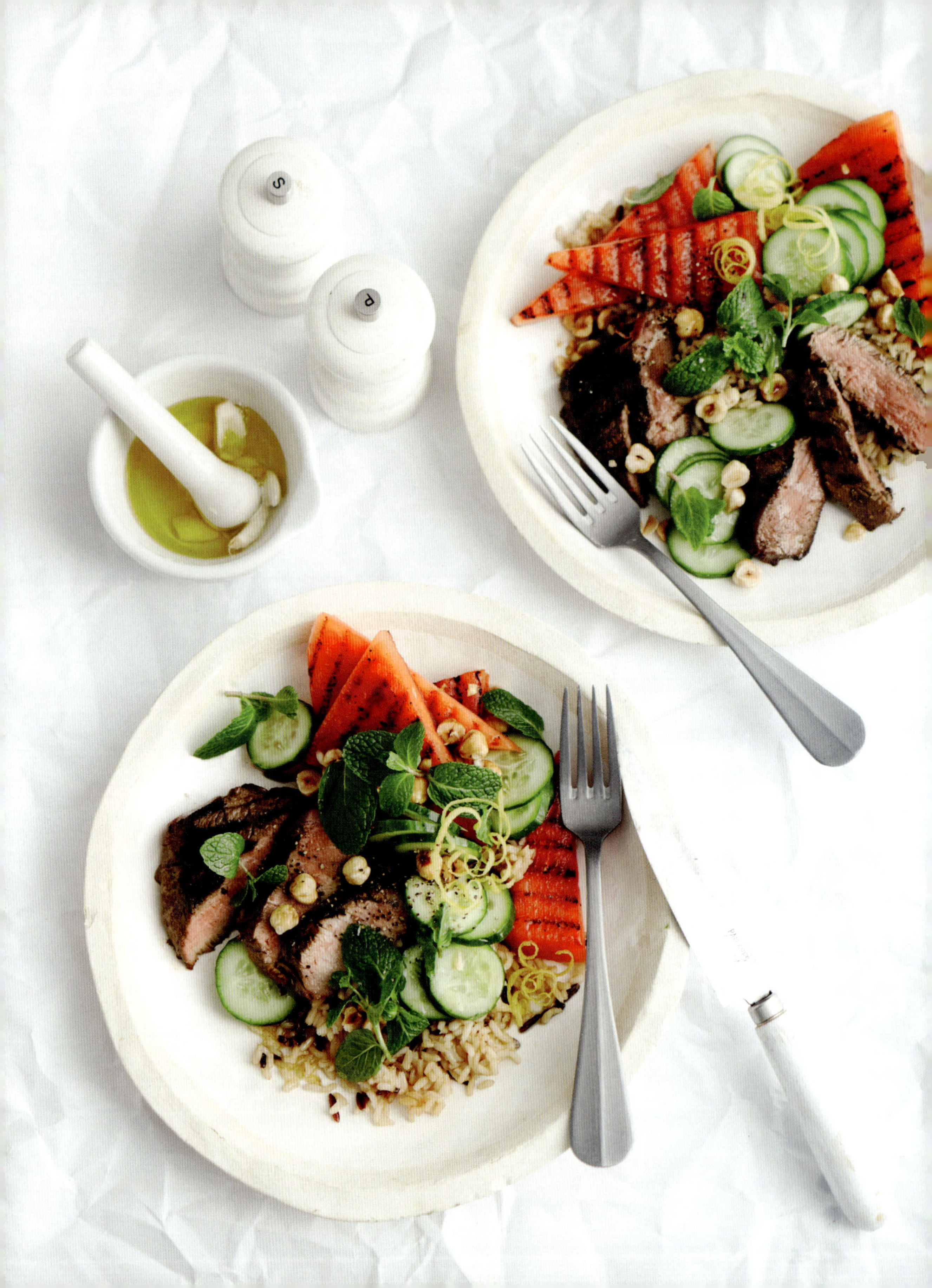
S
P

GRILLED BEEF & WATERMELON SALAD

PREP + COOK TIME *40 MINUTES (+ REFRIGERATION)*
SERVES *4*

2 cloves garlic

⅓ cup (80ml) extra virgin olive oil

1 tbsp honey

4 x 100g beef fillet steaks

½ medium watermelon (1.5kg)

¼ cup (60ml) lemon juice (see tips)

250g microwave brown and wild rice

1 Lebanese cucumber (130g), sliced thinly

1 cup flat-leaf parsley leaves

½ cup mint leaves

⅓ cup (45g) skinless hazelnuts, roasted

1 tbsp thin strips lemon rind (see tips)

1 Thinly slice one garlic clove. Combine 2 tablespoons oil, the honey and sliced garlic in a medium bowl. Add beef; toss to coat. Cover; refrigerate for 1 hour.

2 Meanwhile, remove rind from watermelon. Cut wedge in half lengthways, then into 1cm thick triangles.

3 Preheat a large grill plate (or grill pan) until smoking hot. Grill watermelon, in batches, for 50 seconds each side or until charred lightly. Transfer to a plate; refrigerate for 20 minutes.

4 On a clean grill plate over high heat, cook beef for 3 minutes each side for medium or until cooked to your liking. Transfer to a plate. Cover loosely with foil; rest for 10 minutes, slice thickly.

5 Meanwhile, to make dressing, crush remaining garlic clove. Place the remaining oil, the lemon juice and crushed garlic in a screw-top jar; shake well. Season to taste.

6 Heat rice according to packet directions. Arrange rice on a large platter with watermelon and beef; top with cucumber and herbs. Drizzle with dressing; scatter with hazelnuts and lemon rind.

TIPS It is easier to remove the rind from the lemon before you squeeze the juice. To create the thin strips of lemon rind, use a zester if you have one. If you don't have one, peel two long, wide pieces of rind from the lemon, without the white pith, then cut lengthways into thin strips.

NUTRITION PER SERVING *32.2G TOTAL FAT (5.6G SATURATED FAT); 2509KJ (600 CAL); 44.5G CARBOHYDRATE; 30G PROTEIN; 8.7G FIBRE*

CHORIZO, BLACK BEAN & PUMPKIN SALAD

PREP + COOK TIME *1 HOUR 10 MINUTES*
SERVES *4*

⅓ cup (80ml) extra virgin olive oil

2 tsp ground cumin

2 tsp smoked paprika

2 x 650g kent pumpkins, cut into wedges

1 large red onion (300g), cut into wedges

2 x 125g cured chorizo sausages, sliced thickly

400g can black beans, drained, rinsed

2 long red chillies, sliced thinly

½ cup flat-leaf parsley leaves

½ cup coriander sprigs

SHERRY VINEGAR DRESSING

2 tbsp sherry vinegar

2 tbsp extra virgin olive oil

1 clove garlic, crushed

1 Preheat oven to 200°C. Line a large oven tray with baking paper.

2 Combine oil, half the cumin and half the paprika in a bowl; season. Place pumpkin and onion on lined tray, pour over the spice mixture; turn to coat evenly. Roast for 30 minutes.

3 Combine chorizo, beans and half the chilli in a large bowl with remaining cumin and paprika. Add to tray with pumpkin; cook for a further 20 minutes or until chorizo and pumpkin are browned.

4 Meanwhile, to make sherry vinegar dressing, place ingredients in a screw-top jar; shake well. Season to taste.

5 Layer pumpkin, onion and chorizo mixture on a large platter; drizzle with dressing. Serve topped with parsley, coriander and remaining chilli.

NUTRITION PER SERVING *45.5G TOTAL FAT (10.7G SATURATED FAT); 2870KJ (686 CAL); 39.8G CARBOHYDRATE; 25.2G PROTEIN; 14.9G FIBRE*

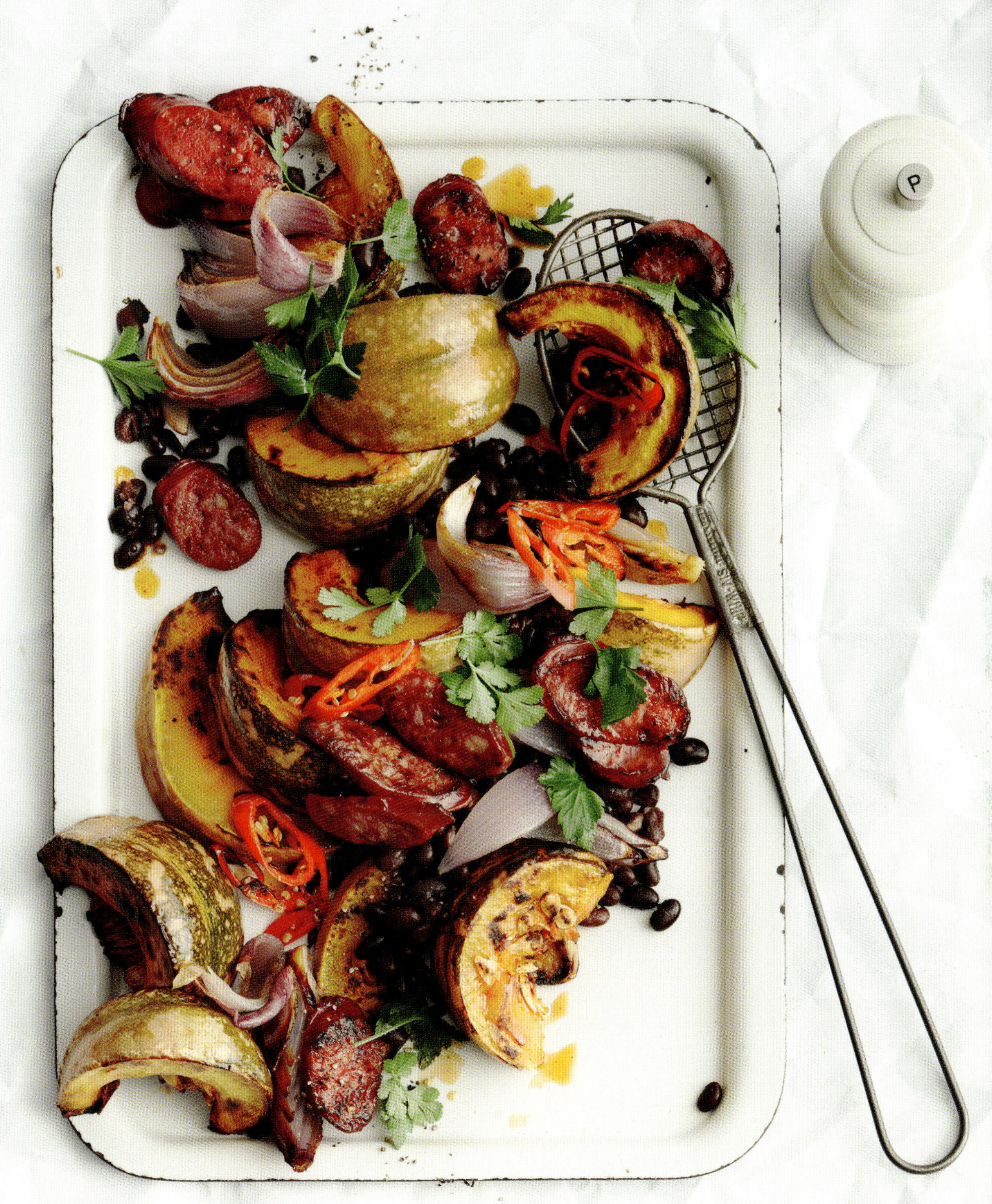
P

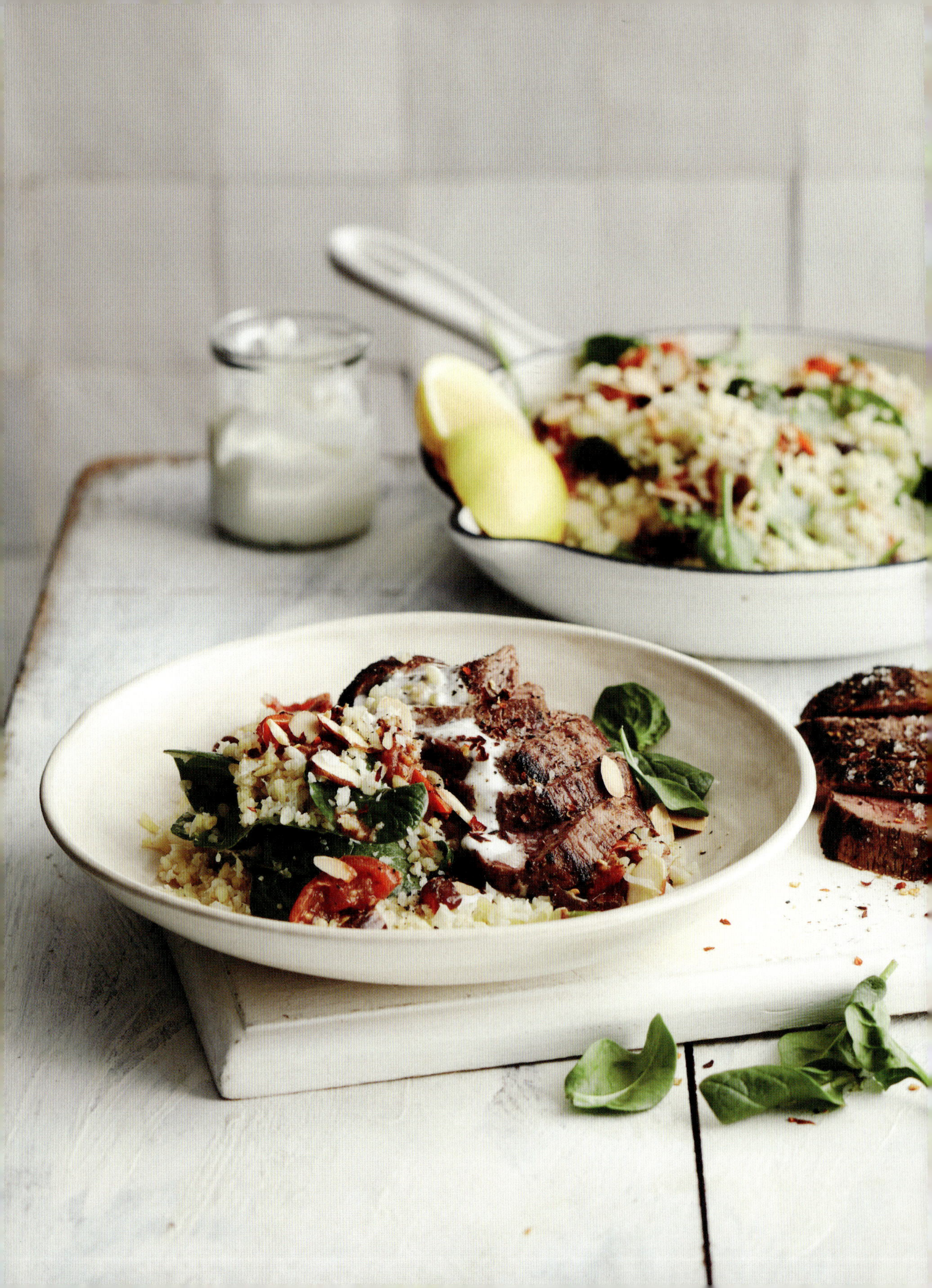

TOMATO & SUMAC LAMB WITH ALMOND BULGUR

PREP + COOK TIME *25 MINUTES (+ STANDING)*
SERVES 4

- **250g cherry tomatoes, chopped coarsely**
- **2 cloves garlic, crushed**
- **2 tsp sumac**
- **¼ cup (60ml) extra virgin olive oil**
- **600g lamb backstraps**
- **1 small cauliflower (1kg), chopped coarsely**
- **1 cup (160g) coarse bulgur wheat**
- **½ cup (60g) natural flaked almonds, roasted**
- **¼ cup (60g) fresh dates, pitted, chopped coarsely**
- **2 tbsp finely chopped coriander**
- **60g baby spinach leaves**
- **½ tsp dried chilli flakes**
- **Greek yoghurt and lemon cheeks, to serve**

1 Combine tomatoes, garlic, sumac and 1 tablespoon of the oil in a large bowl. Add lamb; turn to coat. Cover; stand for 10 minutes.

2 Process cauliflower, in batches, until just coarsely chopped.

3 Heat a large non-stick frying pan over medium-high heat. Remove lamb from bowl, reserving tomato marinade; cook lamb for 4 minutes each side for medium-rare or until cooked to your liking. Rest, loosely covered, for 10 minutes. Wipe frying pan clean; reserve.

4 Meanwhile, place bulgur in a medium bowl. Add enough boiling water to just cover. Cover bowl; stand for 15 minutes until water is absorbed. Drain if necessary.

5 Add reserved tomato marinade and ¼ cup (60ml) water to reserved cleaned pan; cook over medium heat for 2 minutes or until tomato breaks down slightly and mixture is thickened. Transfer to a bowl. Wipe pan clean.

6 Heat remaining 2 tablespoons olive oil in cleaned pan; cook cauliflower, stirring occasionally, for 7 minutes or until softened and beginning to brown. Add tomato marinade and cooked bulgur, then almonds, dates and coriander; toss gently to combine.

7 Top burghul mixture with sliced lamb and spinach leaves; sprinkle with chilli flakes. Serve with dollops of yoghurt and lemon cheeks.

NUTRITION PER SERVING *32.9G TOTAL FAT (6.7G SATURATED FAT); 3214KJ (768 CAL); 55.5G CARBOHYDRATE; 58.5G PROTEIN; 10.8G FIBRE*

MEDITERRANEAN BEEF SALAD

PREP + COOK TIME *25 MINUTES*
SERVES *4*

2 tbsp extra virgin olive oil

1 clove garlic, crushed

1 large red onion (300g), cut into 8 wedges

1 medium eggplant (300g), cut into wedges

1 medium zucchini (120g), halved lengthways

1 medium red capsicum (200g), seeded, quartered

400g can chickpeas, drained, rinsed

200g rare roast beef, torn coarsely (see tip)

100g mixed salad leaves

3 medium roma tomatoes (225g), cut into 8 wedges

OREGANO YOGHURT DRESSING

½ cup (140g) Greek yoghurt

¼ cup oregano leaves, chopped finely

2 tbsp lemon juice

1 tsp finely grated lemon rind

1 Combine oil and garlic in a small bowl; brush onion, eggplant, zucchini and capsicum with garlic oil. Heat a grill plate (or grill pan) over high heat; cook onion, zucchini and capsicum, in batches, for 2 minutes each side, and eggplant for 4 minutes each side or until grill marks appear; transfer to a tray. Cut vegetables into chunks.

2 To make oregano yoghurt dressing, combine ingredients in a bowl. Season to taste.

3 Combine chickpeas, roast beef, salad leaves, tomato and chargrilled vegetables in a large bowl or platter; drizzle with oregano yoghurt dressing. Season to taste.

TIP Rare roast beef can be bought from a delicatessen or the deli counter at major supermarkets.

PREP IT Portion salad and dressing, separately, into airtight containers. Keep refrigerated for up to 4 days.

NUTRITION PER SERVING *13.6G TOTAL FAT (3.2G SATURATED FAT); 1268KJ (303 CAL); 1.7G CARBOHYDRATE; 18.3G PROTEIN; 8.8G FIBRE*

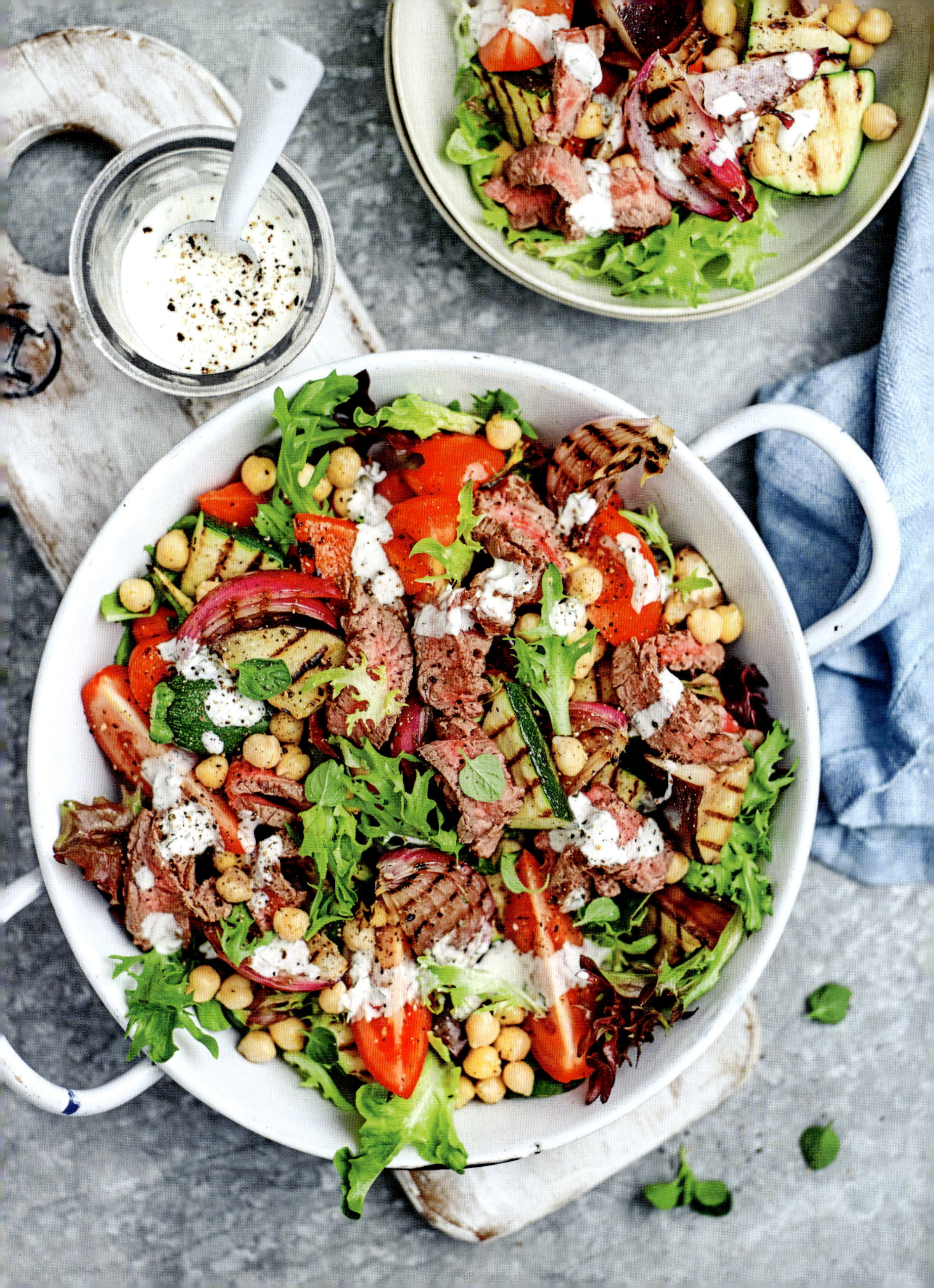

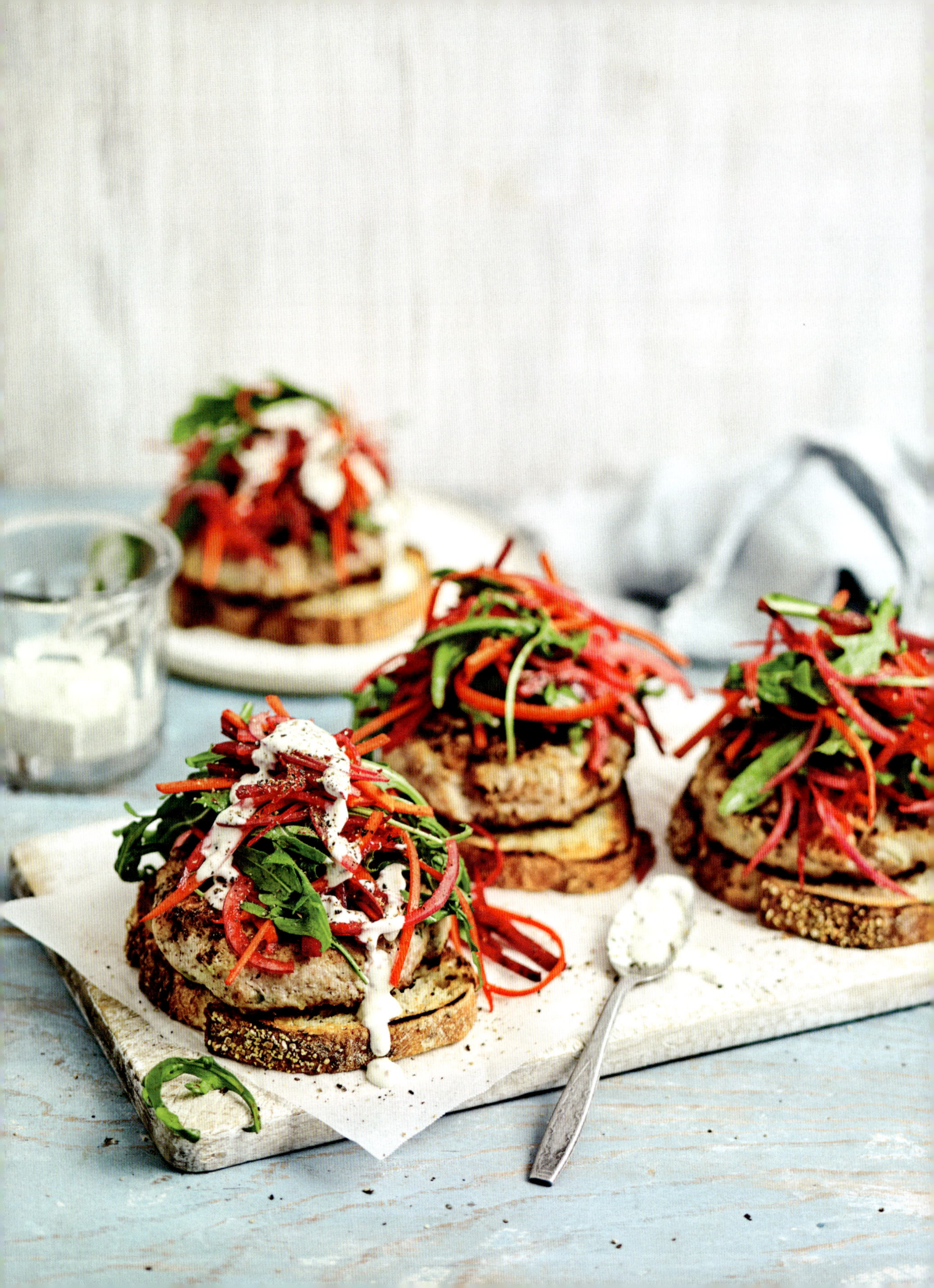

OPEN PORK BURGERS & SLAW

PREP + COOK TIME *40 MINUTES (+ REFRIGERATION)*
SERVES *4*

400g extra-lean minced pork
1 tbsp thyme leaves, chopped finely
1½ tsp ground cumin
1½ tsp ground coriander
1 clove garlic, crushed
1 extra-large egg (60g)
1 small green apple (130g), grated coarsely
400g can cannellini beans, drained, rinsed
olive oil spray
2 tsp apple cider vinegar
¼ tsp finely grated orange rind
2 tsp orange juice
2 tsp extra virgin olive oil
1 cup baby rocket leaves
1 medium carrot (120g), cut into julienne (see tip)
1 medium beetroot (175g), cut into julienne (see tip)
½ small red onion (50g), sliced thinly
4 slices wholegrain bread (120g)

MUSTARD YOGHURT
⅓ cup (95g) Greek yoghurt
3 tsp wholegrain mustard

1 Place pork, thyme, cumin, coriander, garlic, egg, grated apple and beans in a large bowl; mix well. Season. Using wet hands, shape mixture into 4 patties. Cover; refrigerate for 20 minutes to firm.

2 Heat a medium non-stick frying pan over medium heat; spray lightly with oil. Cook burger patties for 6 minutes each side or until cooked through.

3 Meanwhile, to make mustard yoghurt, combine ingredients in a bowl.

4 Combine vinegar, orange rind and juice, and oil in a jug. Toss rocket, carrot, beetroot and onion in a large bowl; drizzle with orange dressing.

5 Lightly toast bread. Top each slice with a burger patty, a quarter of the slaw and a quarter of the mustard yoghurt.

TIP You can coarsely grate the carrot and beetroot instead of julienning them, if you like.

PREP IT Portion patties, mustard yoghurt and undressed slaw separately in airtight containers. Refrigerate for up to 3 days.

NUTRITION PER SERVING *17.9G TOTAL FAT (5.7G SATURATED FAT); 1804KJ (431 CAL); 30.5G CARBOHYDRATE; 31.2G PROTEIN; 9.9G FIBRE*

BEEF TACO SALAD

PREP + COOK TIME *35 MINUTES*
SERVES *4*

- **2 tsp extra virgin olive oil, plus extra to serve**
- **1 large red onion (300g), chopped finely**
- **2 cloves garlic, chopped finely**
- **500g lean beef mince**
- **⅓ cup (95g) tomato paste**
- **30g packet taco seasoning**
- **400g can red kidney beans, drained, rinsed**
- **175g plain corn chips**
- **1 cup (120g) coarsely grated cheddar**
- **2 baby cos lettuce (360g)**
- **250g cherry tomatoes, halved and quartered**
- **1 medium avocado, sliced thinly**
- **½ cup coriander sprigs**
- **lime wedges, to serve**

1 Heat oil in a large frying pan over high heat; cook onion, garlic and beef, stirring, for 5 minutes or until beef is browned.

2 Add tomato paste, seasoning and 1½ cups (375ml) water to beef mixture; stir until well combined. Bring to the boil. Reduce heat to low; simmer for 10 minutes or until most of the liquid has evaporated. Add beans; stir until heated through.

3 Preheat grill to high. Place corn chips, in a single layer, on an oven tray; top with cheese. Place under the grill for 2 minutes or until cheese has melted.

4 Meanwhile, separate outer leaves of lettuce; chop hearts.

5 Divide lettuce, beef mixture and cheesy corn chips among bowls; top with tomatoes, avocado and coriander. Drizzle with extra oil; season with ground pepper. Serve with lime wedges.

NUTRITION PER SERVING *41.4G TOTAL FAT (16.6G SATURATED FAT); 3242KJ (775 CAL); 43.9G CARBOHYDRATE; 47.7G PROTEIN; 15.8G FIBRE*

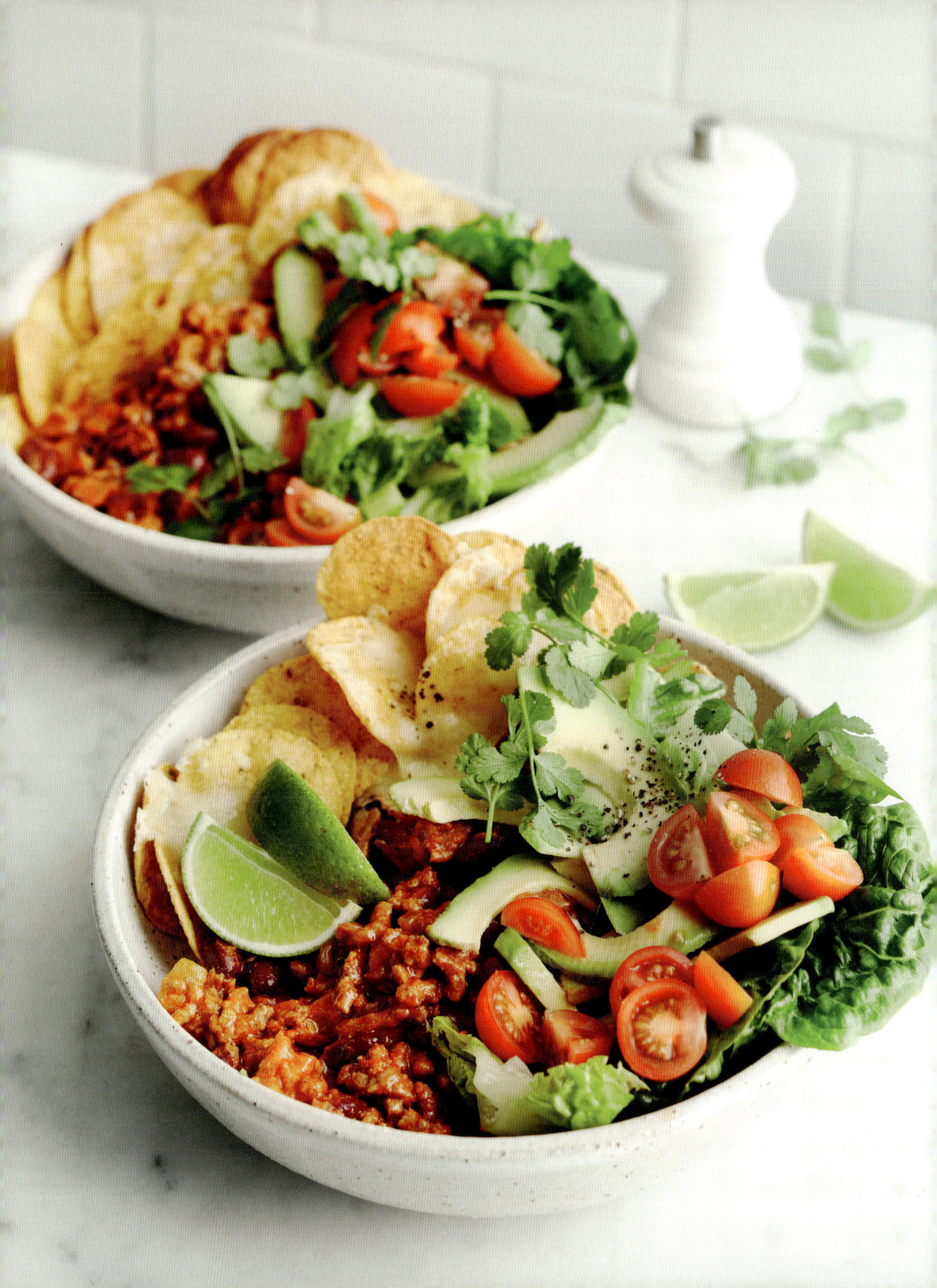

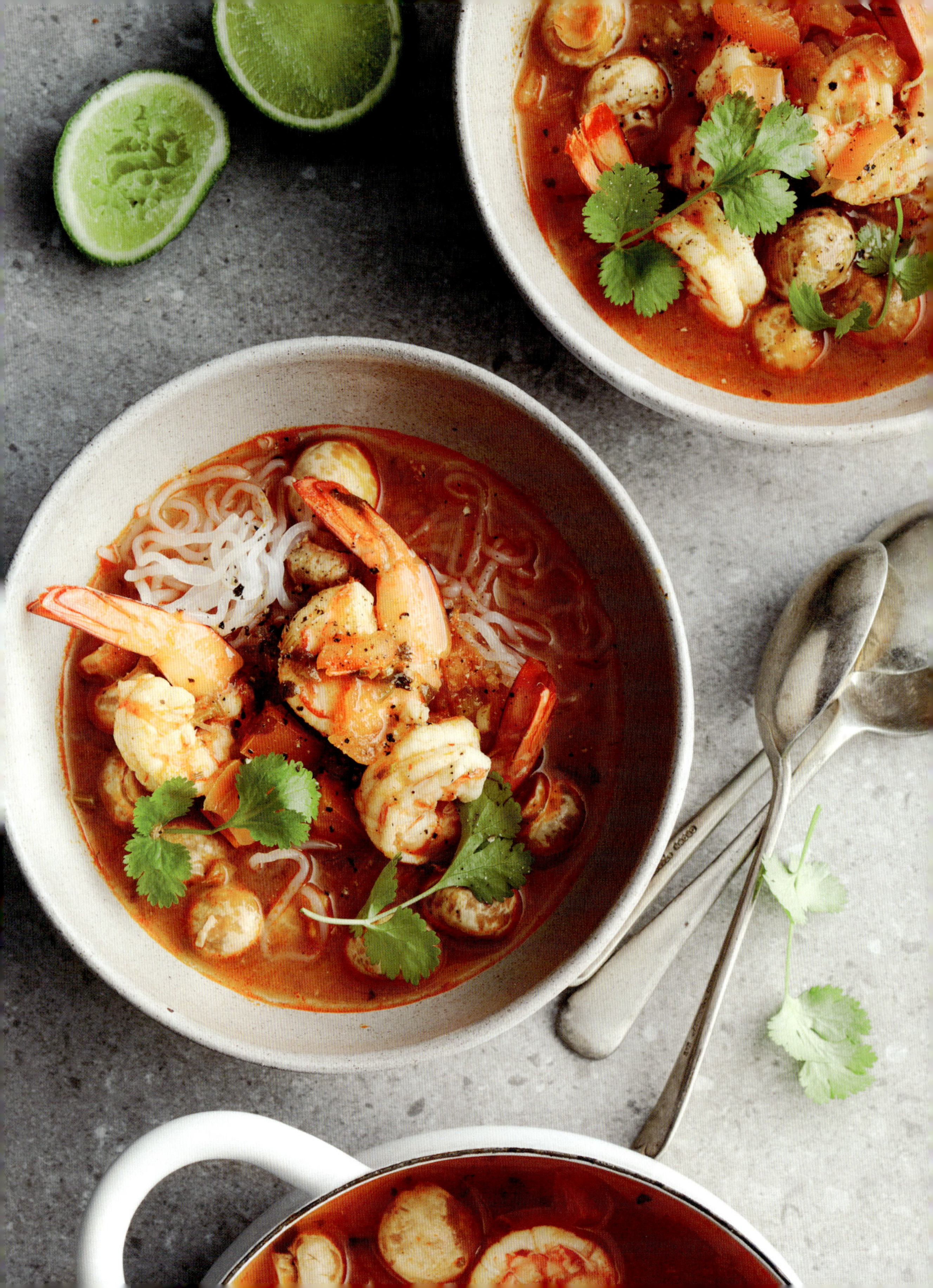

HOT & SOUR SOUP

PREP + COOK TIME *25 MINUTES*
SERVES *4*

- **400g packet konjac noodles (see tip)**
- **1 tbsp extra virgin olive oil**
- **4 green onions, chopped**
- **¼ cup finely chopped coriander leaves and stems, plus ½ cup extra leaves, to serve**
- **2 tbsp tom yum paste**
- **1 litre (4 cups) fish stock**
- **10cm stalk lemongrass, bruised**
- **1 tbsp tamarind puree**
- **20 uncooked prawns (900g), peeled, deveined with tails intact**
- **200g button mushrooms**
- **2 medium tomatoes (300g), chopped**
- **2 tbps lime juice**
- **lime cheeks, to serve**

1 Drain noodles from packet liquid; place in a heatproof bowl. Cover with boiling water; stand for 1 minute, drain well.

2 Heat oil in a large saucepan; cook green onion and chopped coriander for 1 minute until softened. Add tom yum paste; cook, stirring, for 30 seconds. Add stock, lemongrass and tamarind; bring to the boil. Reduce heat; cook for 5 minutes.

3 Stir in prawns, mushrooms and tomato; cook for 5 minutes or until prawns are cooked through. Stir in lime juice.

4 Divide noodles among bowls; ladle soup over noodles. Serve topped with extra coriander leaves and lime cheeks.

TIP Konjac noodles are made from the vegetable Konjac and are famed for their low-kilojoules and low carbohydrate content. They are available from major supermarkets.

NUTRITION PER SERVING *9.4G TOTAL FAT (2.4G SATURATED FAT); 1109KJ (265 CAL); 14.4G CARBOHYDRATE; 27.6G PROTEIN; 8.5G FIBRE*

GLOSSARY

ALMONDS flat, pointy-tipped nuts having a pitted brown shell enclosing a creamy white kernel which is covered by a brown skin.
flaked paper-thin slices.
BAKING POWDER a raising agent consisting mainly of two parts cream of tartar to one part bicarbonate of soda.
BEANS
black also called turtle beans or black kidney beans; an earthy-flavoured dried bean. Used mostly in Mexican and South American cooking.
black-eyed also called black-eyed peas or cow peas. Mild-flavoured and thin-skinned, so they cook faster than most other beans.
cannellini small white bean similar in flavour and appearance to other phaseolus vulgaris varieties (great northern, navy or haricot).
green also called French or string beans (although the tough string they once had has generally been bred out of them), this long thin bean is consumed in its entirety once cooked.
kidney medium-size red bean, slightly floury in texture yet sweet in flavour; sold dried or canned, it's found in bean mixes and is used in chilli con carne.
sprouts tender new growths of assorted beans and seeds germinated for consumption as sprouts.
BICARBONATE OF SODA a raising agent.
BULGUR also called burghul; hulled steamed wheat kernels that, once dried, are crushed into various-sized grains. Used in Middle-Eastern dishes such as falafel, kibbeh and tabbouleh. Is not the same as cracked wheat.
CARDAMOM a spice native to India and used extensively in its cuisine; can be purchased in pod, seed or ground form.
CHEESE
fetta Greek in origin; a crumbly textured goat's- or sheep-milk cheese with a sharp, salty taste. Ripened and stored in salted whey.
mozzarella soft, spun-curd cheese; originating in southern Italy where it was traditionally made from water-buffalo milk. Now generally made from cow's milk, it is the most popular pizza cheese because of its low melting point and elasticity when heated.
paneer a simple, delicate fresh cheese used as a major source of protein in the Indian diet.
parmesan also called parmigiano; is a hard, grainy cow's-milk cheese originating in Italy. Reggiano is the best variety.
ricotta a soft, sweet, moist, white cow's-milk cheese with a low fat content (8.5%) and a slightly grainy texture. The name roughly translates as 'cooked again' and refers to ricotta's manufacture from a whey that is itself a by-product of other cheese making.
CHIA SEEDS contain protein and all the essential amino acids and a wealth of vitamins, minerals and antioxidants, as well as being fibre-rich.
CHICKPEAS also called hummus or channa; an irregularly round, sandy-coloured legume. Has a firm texture, even after cooking, a floury mouth-feel and a robust nutty flavour; available canned or dried.
CORIANDER also known as pak chee or chinese parsley; a bright-green leafy herb with a pungent flavour. Both stems and roots of coriander are also used in cooking; wash well before using. Also available ground or as seeds; these should not be substituted for fresh as the tastes are completely different.
COUSCOUS a fine, grain-like cereal product made from semolina; from North Africa.
CUMIN also called zeera or comino; resembling caraway in size, cumin is the dried seed of a plant related to the parsley family. Available dried as seeds or ground.
EDAMAME (SHELLED SOYBEANS) available frozen from Asian food stores and some supermarkets.
FENNEL also called finocchio or anise; a white to very pale green-white, firm, crisp, roundish vegetable. The bulb has a slightly sweet, anise flavour but the feathery fronds have a much stronger taste.

FISH SAUCE also called nam pla or nuoc nam; made from pulverised salted fermented fish, most often anchovies. Has a pungent smell and strong taste, so use sparingly.

FIVE-SPICE POWDER although the ingredients vary from country to country, five-spice is usually a fragrant mixture of ground cinnamon, cloves, star anise, Sichuan pepper and fennel seeds. Used in Chinese and other Asian cooking; available from most supermarkets or Asian food shops.

FLOUR

plain unbleached wheat flour; is the best for baking as the gluten content ensures a strong dough for a light result.

self-raising plain all-purpose flour sifted with baking powder in the proportion of 1 cup flour to 2 teaspoons baking powder.

wholemeal also known as wholewheat flour; milled with the wheat germ so is higher in fibre and more nutritional than plain flour.

HORSERADISH CREAM a commercially prepared creamy paste consisting of grated horseradish, vinegar, oil and sugar.

KALE a type of leafy cabbage, rich in nutrients and vitamins. Leaf colours can range from green to violet.

LENTILS (red, brown, yellow) dried pulses often identified by and named after their colour; also known as dhal.

LINSEEDS also known as flaxseed, they are the richest plant source of omega 3 fats, which are essential for a healthy brain, heart, joints and immune system.

MAKRUT LIME LEAVES also known as bai magrood and looks like two glossy dark green leaves joined end to end, forming a rounded hourglass shape. Used fresh or dried in many South-East Asian dishes; dried leaves are less potent so double the number if substituting for fresh. A strip of fresh lime peel may be substituted for each makrut lime leaf.

MAPLE SYRUP distilled from the sap of sugar maple trees. Maple-flavoured syrup or pancake syrup is not an substitute for the real thing.

MAYONNAISE, WHOLE-EGG commercial mayonnaise of high quality made with whole eggs and labelled as such; some prepared mayonnaises substitute emulsifiers such as food starch, cellulose gel or other thickeners to achieve the same thick and creamy consistency but never achieve the same rich flavour. Must be refrigerated once opened.

MIRIN a Japanese champagne-coloured cooking wine; made of glutinous rice and alcohol and used expressly for cooking. Should not be confused with sake.

MISO fermented soybean paste. There are many types of miso, each with its own aroma, flavour, colour and texture; it can be kept, airtight, for up to a year in the fridge. The darker the miso, the saltier the taste and denser the texture.

MIXED SPICE a classic spice mixture generally containing caraway, allspice, coriander, cumin, nutmeg and ginger, although cinnamon and other spices can be added. It is used with fruit and in cakes.

NORI a type of dried seaweed used in Japanese cooking as a flavouring, garnish or for sushi. Sold in thin sheets, plain or toasted (yaki-nori).

OIL

cooking spray we use a cholesterol-free cooking spray made from canola oil; a 1-second spray equals 1g fat.

olive made from ripened olives. Extra virgin and virgin are the first and second press, respectively, of the olives and are therefore considered the best; the 'extra light' or 'light' name refers to taste, not fat levels.

sesame made from roasted, crushed, white sesame seeds; a flavouring rather than a cooking medium.

ONIONS

eschalot also called French shallots or golden shallots. Small and elongated, with a brown skin, they grow in tight clusters similar to garlic.

green also known, incorrectly, as shallots; an immature onion picked before the bulb has formed, having a long, bright-green edible stalk.

red also known as Spanish, red Spanish or Bermuda onion; a sweet-flavoured, large, purple-red onion.
PAPRIKA ground dried sweet red capsicum; there are many grades and types available, including sweet, hot, mild and smoked.
QUINOA (pronounced keen-wa) is cooked and eaten as a grain alternative, but is in fact a seed. It has a delicate, nutty taste and chewy texture, and is gluten free.
flakes the grains have been rolled and flattened.
RADICCHIO Italian in origin; a member of the chicory family. The dark burgundy leaves and strong, bitter flavour can be cooked or eaten raw in salads.
ROSEWATER extract made from crushed rose petals, called gulab in India; used for its aromatic quality in desserts.
SESAME SEEDS black and white are the most common of this small oval seed, however there are also red and brown varieties.
SUGAR
caster finely granulated table sugar.
palm also called nam tan pip, jaggery, jawa or gula melaka; made from the sap of the sugar palm tree.
SUMAC a purple-red, astringent spice ground from berries growing on shrubs flourishing wild around the Mediterranean; adds a tart, lemony flavour to food. Available from supermarkets.
TAHINI sesame seed paste available from Middle Eastern food stores and supermarkets.
TAMARI similar to but thicker than Japanese soy; very dark in colour with a distinctively mellow flavour. Good used as a dipping sauce or for basting. Some brands are gluten free.
TOFU also known as soybean curd or bean curd; an off-white, custard-like product made from the 'milk' of crushed soybeans.
firm made by compressing bean curd to remove most of the water.
silken not a type of tofu but reference to the manufacturing process of straining soybean liquid through silk; this denotes best quality.
TURMERIC also called kamin; is a rhizome related to galangal and ginger. Fresh turmeric can be substituted with the more commonly found dried powder. When fresh turmeric is called for in a recipe, the dried powder can be substituted (1 teaspoon of ground turmeric for every 20g of fresh turmeric).
VINEGAR
balsamic originally from Modena, Italy, there are now many balsamic vinegars on the market ranging in pungency and quality depending on how long they have been aged. Is a deep rich brown colour and has a sweet and sour flavour.
red wine based on fermented red wine.
rice a colourless vinegar made from fermented rice, sugar and salt.
white wine made from white wine.
white made from distilled grain alcohol.
VANILLA
bean dried, long, thin pod from a tropical golden orchid; the minuscule black seeds inside the bean are used to impart a luscious vanilla flavour in baking and desserts.
bean paste made from vanilla beans and contains real seeds. Is highly concentrated: 1 teaspoon replaces a whole vanilla bean. Found in supermarkets in the baking section.
extract obtained from vanilla beans infused in water; a non-alcoholic version of essence.
WATERCRESS one of the cress family, a large group of peppery greens used raw in salads, dips and sandwiches, or cooked in soups. Highly perishable, so it must be used as soon as possible after purchase.
WOMBOK also known as Chinese cabbage or Peking cabbage; elongated in shape with pale green, crinkly leaves, this is the most common cabbage in South-East Asia.
ZA'ATAR a Middle Eastern herb and spice mixture which varies; always includes thyme, with ground sumac and, usually, toasted sesame seeds.
ZUCCHINI also known as courgette; belongs to the squash family. Yellow flowers can be stuffed or used in salads.

CONVERSION CHART

MEASURES

One Australian metric measuring cup holds approximately 250ml; one Australian metric tablespoon holds 20ml; one Australian metric teaspoon holds 5ml.

The difference between one country's measuring cups and another's is within a two- or three-teaspoon variance, and will not affect your cooking results. North America, New Zealand and the United Kingdom use a 15ml tablespoon. All cup and spoon measurements are level.

The most accurate way of measuring dry ingredients is to weigh them.

When measuring liquids, use a clear glass or plastic jug with the metric markings.

We use extra-large eggs with an average weight of 60g.

DRY MEASURES

metric	imperial
15g	½oz
30g	1oz
60g	2oz
90g	3oz
125g	4oz (¼lb)
155g	5oz
185g	6oz
220g	7oz
250g	8oz (½lb)
280g	9oz
315g	10oz
345g	11oz
375g	12oz (¾lb)
410g	13oz
440g	14oz
470g	15oz
500g	16oz (1lb)
750g	24oz (1½lb)
1kg	32oz (2lb)

LIQUID MEASURES

metric	imperial
30ml	1 fluid oz
60ml	2 fluid oz
100ml	3 fluid oz
125ml	4 fluid oz
150ml	5 fluid oz
190ml	6 fluid oz
250ml	8 fluid oz
300ml	10 fluid oz
500ml	16 fluid oz
600ml	20 fluid oz
1000ml (1 litre)	1¾ pints

LENGTH MEASURES

metric	imperial
3mm	⅛in
6mm	¼in
1cm	½in
2cm	¾in
2.5cm	1in
5cm	2in
6cm	2½in
8cm	3in
10cm	4in
13cm	5in
15cm	6in
18cm	7in
20cm	8in
22cm	9in
25cm	10in
28cm	11in
30cm	12in (1ft)

OVEN TEMPERATURES

The oven temperatures in this book are for conventional ovens; if you have a fan-forced oven, decrease the temperature by 10-20 degrees.

	°C (Celsius)	°F (Fahrenheit)
Very slow	120	250
Slow	150	300
Moderately slow	160	325
Moderate	180	350
Moderately hot	200	400
Hot	220	425
Very hot	240	475

INDEX

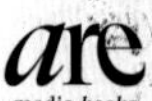

Published in 2022 by Are Media Books, Australia.
Are Media Books is a division of Are Media Pty Ltd.

ARE MEDIA
Chief Executive Officer
Jane Huxley

ARE MEDIA BOOKS
Group Publisher Nicole Byers
Editorial & Food Director
Sophia Young

Books Director David Scotto
Creative Director
Hannah Blackmore
Managing Editor Stephanie Kistner
Designer Dana Brown
Editor Amanda Lees
Food Editor Bronwen Clark

Cover Photographers
John Paul Urizar, Craig Wall
Cover Stylist Kate Brown
Cover Photochef Rebecca Lyall

Printed in China by 1010 Printing International.

A catalogue record for this book is available from the National Library of Australia.
ISBN 978-1-92586-681-0

Published by Are Media Books, a division of Are Media Pty Limited, 54 Park St, Sydney; GPO Box 4088, Sydney, NSW 2001, Australia
Ph +61 2 9282 8000
www.awwcookbooks.com.au

International rights enquiries
internationalrights@aremedia.com.au

Order books
phone 1300 322 007 (within Australia)
or order online at
www.awwcookbooks.com.au

Send recipe enquiries to
recipeenquiries@aremedia.com.au

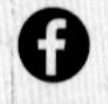 womensweeklyfood

 @womensweeklyfood